QUEER KY

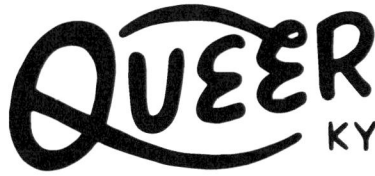

Queer Kentucky is a diverse LGBTQ+ run non-profit based in Kentucky working to bolster and enhance Queer culture and health through storytelling, education, and action. Through our storytelling approach, we give visibility and celebrate the lives of LGBTQ+ people in the great Bluegrass State. Visibility alone is life-saving. Queer Kentucky actively works with organizations and businesses on their inclusivity efforts that enhance the well-being of their employees.

Dedication
To every queer person struggling, and to all those that have succumbed to their struggles.
Please know you aren't alone.

And to the thriving LGBTQ+ people and allies working to enhance the lives of our community.

We see you fighting, and we're standing with you.

DONATE/SUBSCRIBE

QUEER KY

Executive Director
Missy Spears

Editor-in-Chief
Spencer Jenkins

Associate Editor
Hallie Decker

Design
Hannah Schiller,
Brackish Creative

Contributing photographers and artists
Alexia Harris
Andy Mendoza
Lane Levitch
Anthony Munger
Faulkner Morgan Archive
Bearykah Shaw
Josh Drake
Cam Whaley
Simone Jackson
Xander Jarvis
Kyle Angel
Brett Loudermilk
Jon Cherry
Jack Manion
Jacob Grant
Levi House

Contributing writers
Steven Carr
Kevin Garner
Luis Ignacio Andrade
Austyn Gaffney
Joshua Brown
Ashlee Martinis
Tom Lally
Shepherd

Web development
An Agency
Honeywick

*For advertising inquiries
contact@queerkentucky.com*

CONTENTS

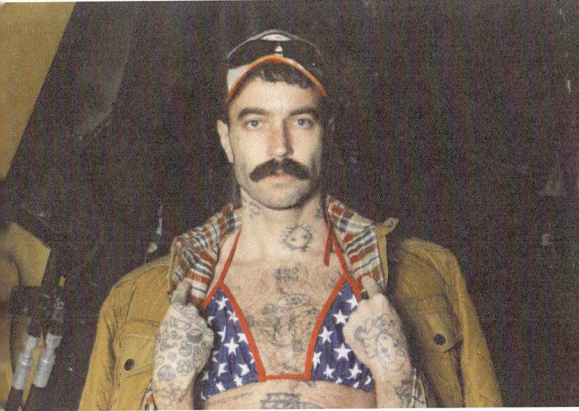

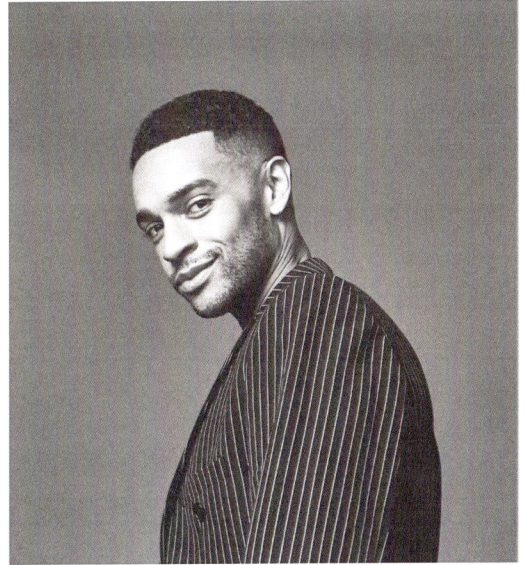

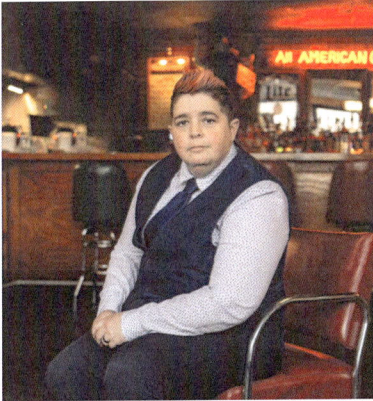

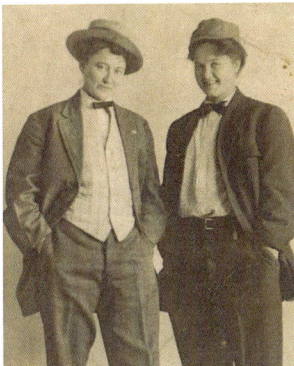

> *"I love being gay. I love spending twenty minutes moisturizing. I love carrying my phone in my hand like a little coin purse. I love poppers. I love incense. I love drama. I love starting phone calls with GIRL and biiiiiitch. I love songs that are just one command, like DANCE, spoken over and over again by a mean Australian lady with cunty bangs. I love crossing my legs, tequila sunrises, and when the bartender calls me 'baby.'"*
>
> Edgar Gomez, "I Love Being Gay"

Dear reader,

Until this flash essay was read to me by my dear friend Minda Honey, I could never quite grasp why I loved being gay so much. I could never find the words to describe why "gay" was my reason for life, but maybe it's because the experiences we share can never properly be put into just one sentence.

Oftentimes as gay men, we are asked, "Why is being gay your whole personality?" This question once brought me unshakeable shame. "There's more to you than being gay, right? Can't you talk about something else?"

I understand that I don't need to explain to people every day that *ARTPOP* is Gaga's most underrated album or detail why I prefer Jungle Juice poppers over RUSH, but even the most mundane energy exchange will be laced with unavoidable queerness any time I open my mouth. My Kentucky-valley girl drawl and my big bashful eyelashes make my responses to oh-so-hetero small talk drip in the deepest degree of gay.

Is there more to me? Am I *too* much? Am I *not enough?* Do I *want* there to be more? As a gay man, I started asking myself these questions when my natural feminine tendencies and traits were called into question — because that's what was really happening.

What I have realized is that my confidence can create uncomfortable feelings in others, but my god-given femininity is everything and something to be proud of. It's my sparkle and my strength that societal norms and the morality police have tried beating out of me over and over again.

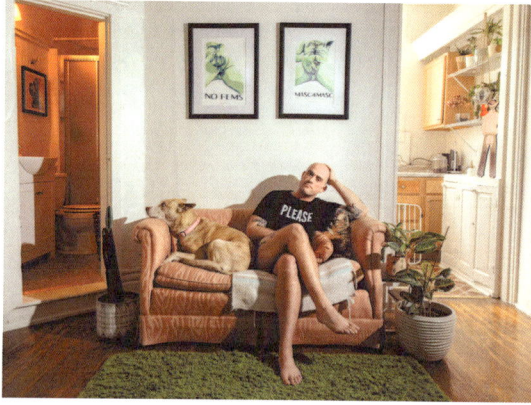

And believe me, I tried conforming to "moral" standards. I tried throwing without a limp wrist. I tried deepening my voice. I tried dating and fucking girls. I tried praying. I tried begging. I did the research and read our culture's imaginary textbook on "how to be a manly man", but every time I took its open-book test I failed. A big ole' F for faggot.

When Minda read this flash essay to me, I think she thought it was a cute, quirky piece for me to connect with because I am always looking for new ways to connect with my queerness. This is true, but she more importantly handed me a blueprint for gay self-love. A Rosetta Stone of sorts for translating why being gay is so amazing.

Every time I wrap up an issue of Queer Kentucky, I wonder how the words between the pages will affect you, dear reader. Will witnessing men in dresses help validate you? Can visible top surgery scars of another make you feel less alone? I hope that these gender-bending Bluegrass stories provide affirming words and phrases that instill pride and joy. I hope as Editor-in-Chief, I can be your Minda and that this magazine works like Edgar's words worked for me.

Love,

photos by Jon Cherry   he/him   @jonpcherry
artwork by Rob Fischer   he/him   @versace_rob

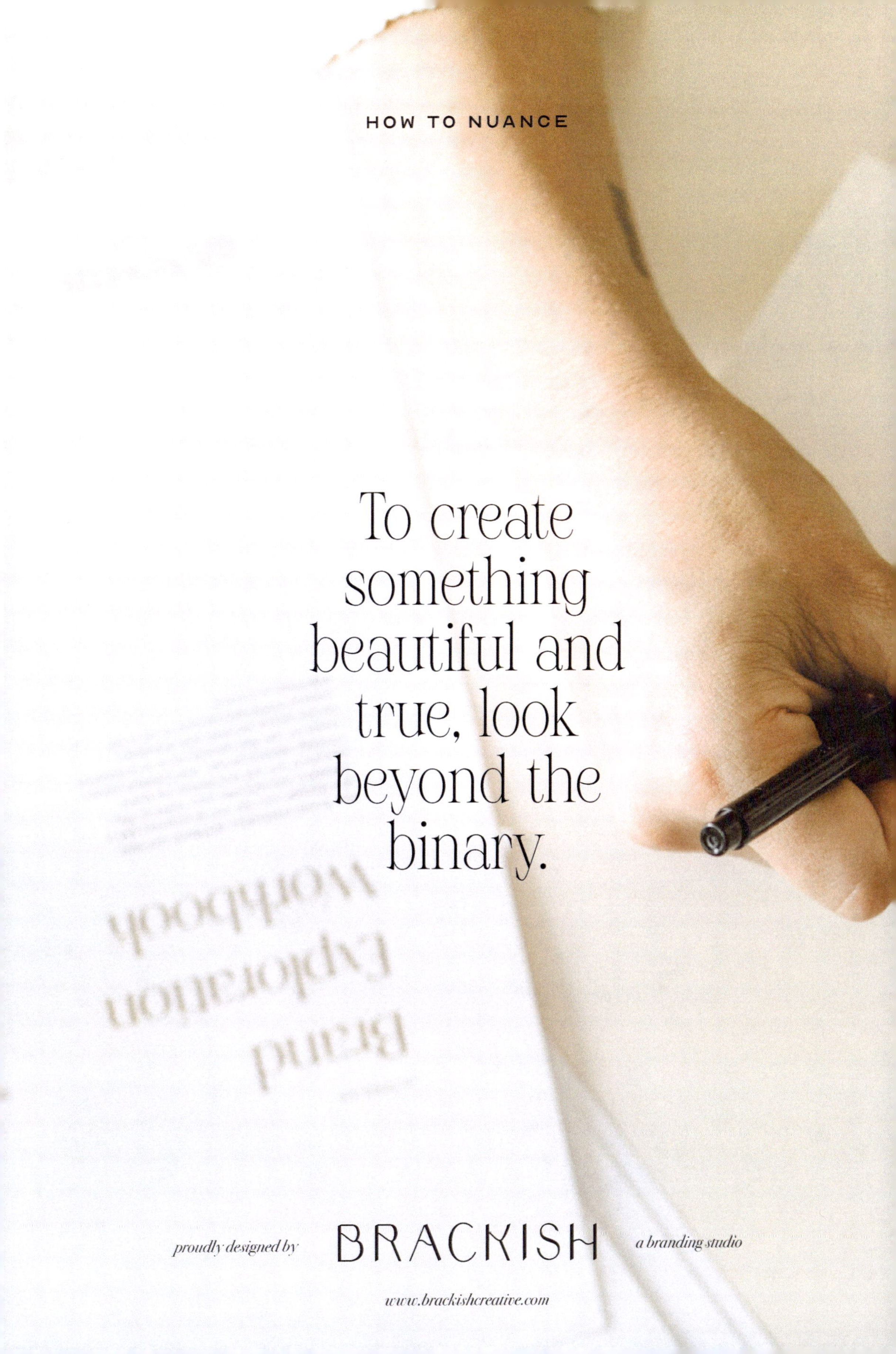

To create
something
beautiful and
true, look
beyond the
binary.

proudly designed by BRACKISH *a branding studio*

www.brackishcreative.com

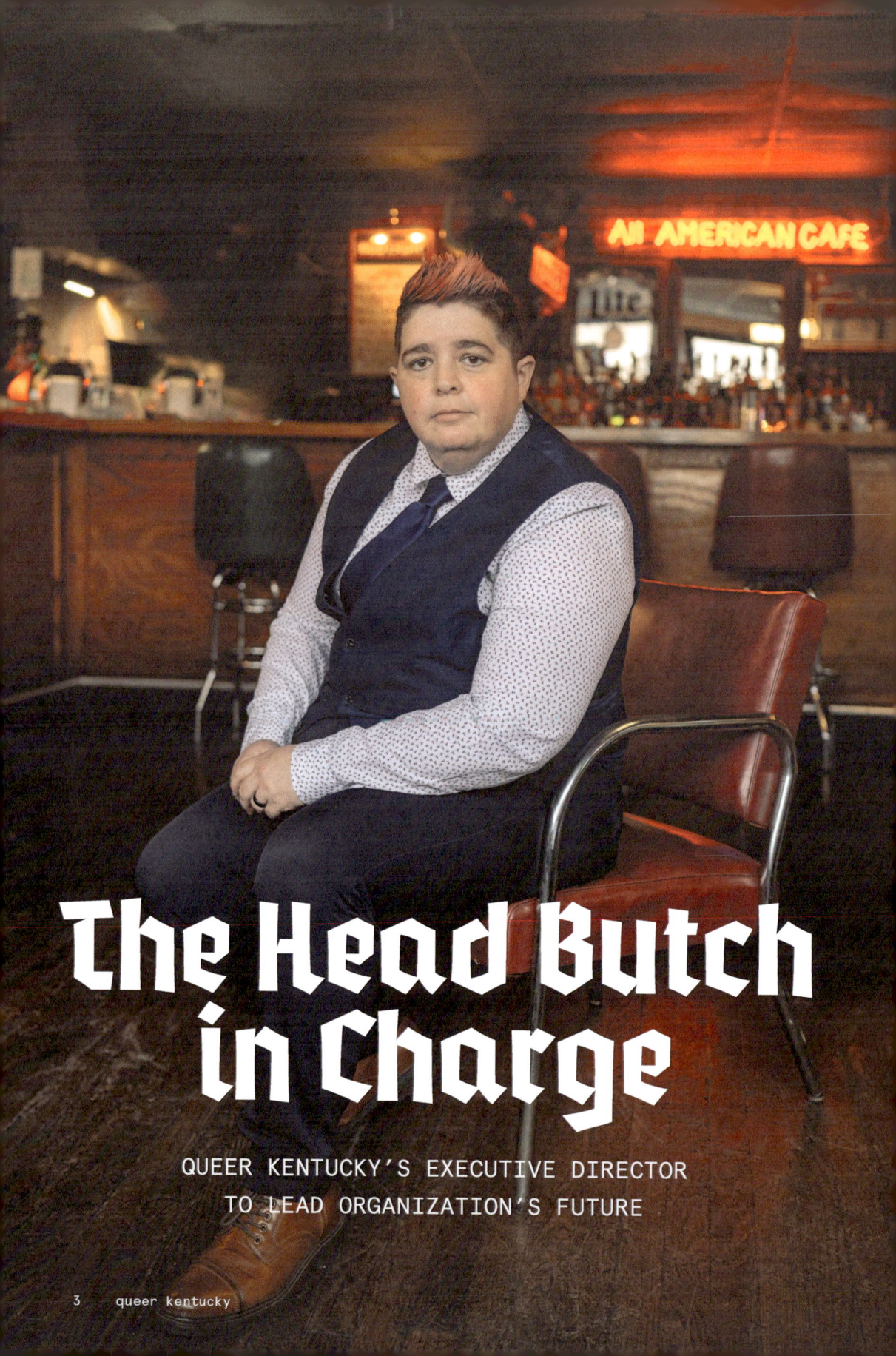

The Head Butch in Charge

QUEER KENTUCKY'S EXECUTIVE DIRECTOR TO LEAD ORGANIZATION'S FUTURE

Missy Spears *she/they* *@missy.spears*

Before I understood queerness, I understood masculinity. When I was a child I emulated masculine stereotypes at every turn: grabbing a hammer I could barely hold to help on a project my dad was working on; wearing my cousin David's corduroy suit to kindergarten; using the bubbles from the bath to form a foam beard around my tiny jaw: doing anything and every-thing to show off in front of a girl. I knew I was different than other girls, but it wasn't until my mom asked me at age seven, after finding a piece of paper on which I had written "I love Alison," over and over again in the perfect cursive I was practicing, if I was gay that I had a term to describe myself. Without being told what the word meant, I immediately knew I was gay. And I immediately knew to hide it.

Never in a million years would that scared, isolated, seven-year-old imag-ine that this would be their life. Married to an incredible woman. Openly queer. Accepted. Loved. And running a quickly growing storytelling-based nonprofit focused on the LGBTQ+ community.

It feels weird introducing myself to you because I feel like I already know you. I'm a 44-year-old Queer that calls Kentucky home. Pink hair. Masculine clothes. Big dreams. Bigger mouth. Neurodivergent. Mentally ill. Former food stamp recipient. College dropout. And I'm the new Executive Director of Queer Kentucky.

I'm a huge proponent of community building by creating spaces that are inviting to the folks most often left on the sidelines. I believe that inclusivity is an intentional action, and that tools like authenticity, storytelling, grass-roots marketing, and the word "fuck" are too often underutilized. And I believe that we don't need approval to do things. Half of the projects on my resume are because I got mad and just did something. Too many stray cats getting hit by cars? Create a trap, neuter, release program called "Cut Your Balls Off Covington." White supremacists putting up recruiting stickers in your neighborhood? Organize your neighbors to identify and remove the propaganda. Gentrification increasing food insecurity around you? Co-found a free fridge program on private property.

I am so grateful to Queer Kentucky's founder Spencer Jenkins for creating and growing such an incredible organization, and I am excited that he has moved into the Editor-in-Chief position, now able to use his journalism skills full time on our web-based and print editorial content. We have so much still left to show you this year, including two more magazines that we've been working on since January, and we are excited for where the organiza-tion is heading.

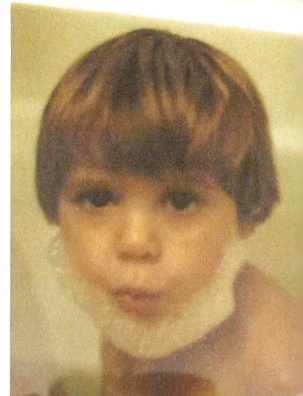

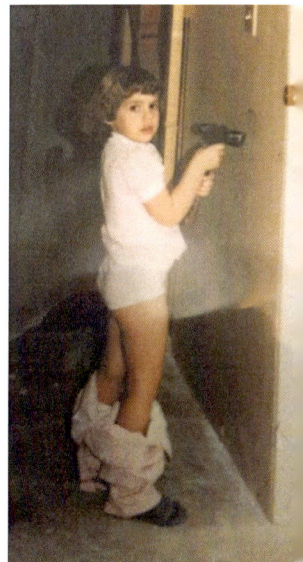

I realize that there is a lot of responsibility in this position and that as I report to my board, I also report to you. You are what makes this organization great. Your stories. Your passion. Your ability to pinpoint and call out bullshit. Your ability to love and offer forgiveness. I look forward to getting to know so many of you through my work at Queer Kentucky, but also through simply being one of you.

Let's Fucking Go

CREATE COMMUNITY AND BECOME CENTERED AT SUSPEND LOUISVILLE.

Mindful Movement is a body inclusive practice designed by queer people, for queer people. Free and open to all.

Sundays 10 - 10:50 a.m.

721 E Washington St, Louisville, KY 40202

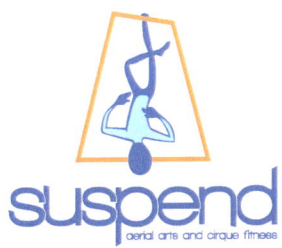

suspend
aerial arts and cirque fitness

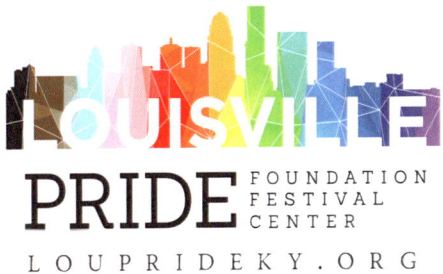

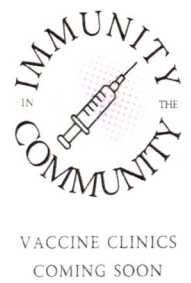

MASCULINITY THROUGH A QUEER [CAMERA] LENS

Alexia Harris   *she/her*   *@lunartheoryofficial*

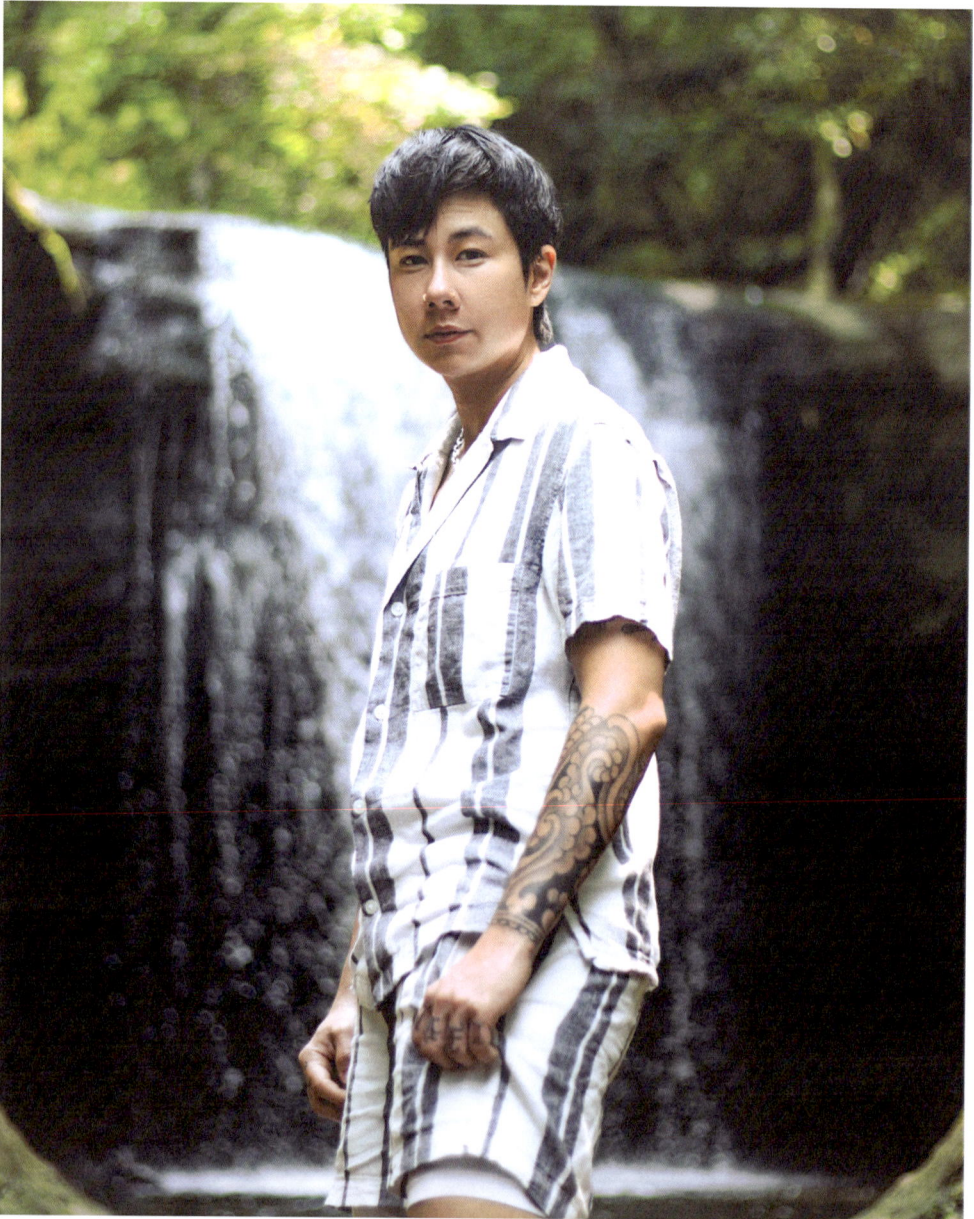

Ashton Kim   *he/they*

photos by Alexia Harris   *she/her*   *@lunartheoryofficial*

It's a complex question that traverses the realms of politics, media, and personal identity. In today's world, where male lawmakers legislate against women's bodies and entire American cities are banning queerness in public, masculinity can feel overwhelmingly like an oppressive force. However, amidst this narrative, masculinity can sometimes also symbolize rebellion, strength, and provide a unique kind of safety. As a photographer, that is something I strive to portray in my work.

When I came out in high school, and during the years that followed, I immersed myself in queer culture and met a vast array of beautiful, diverse, talented people. However, the more queer people I met, and the more time I spent with them, the more obvious it became to me that I didn't see this vibrant community—especially masculine women like the ones I dated- reflected anywhere when I watched TV, read magazines, or looked at art. I knew right away that I wanted to change that.

They say if you want to know what someone loves, look at what they photograph.

From the time I was old enough to hold one, I just about always had a camera in my hand, so it was no surprise that my love letter to the queer community plays out in the form of photography. I started photographing the masculine lesbians I knew at 16-years-old, and as I've gotten older and our language as queer people has expanded, so has my portfolio. Looking through it now, you'll find people who identify as trans-masc, masculine and feminine lesbians, enbies, gender fluid, and a myriad of other identities and expressions. It's a project 20 years in the making and not ending anytime soon.

The decision, as someone other than a cis-het male, to embrace your masculinity with confidence in a world that expects and demands femininity and demureness from you is an act of courage.

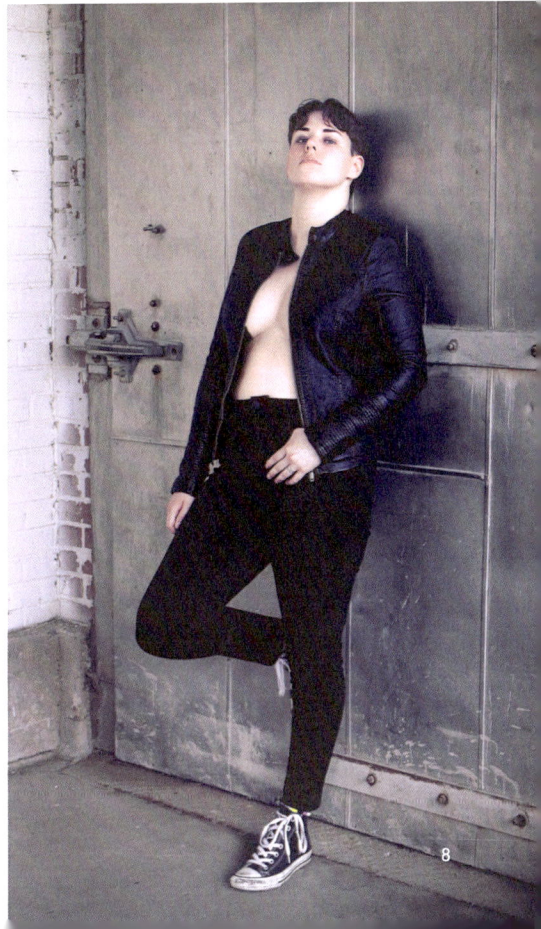

Oriana Ireland   she/her   Shadow Waterson   she/they
Emma McCullough   they/she

8

Slipknot made me GAY

HOW GRUNGE MUSIC BROKE DOWN MY CLOSET DOOR

Steven Carr   *he/him   @thapicklequeen*

Now, I know what you're thinking: Slipknot? Not Britney Spears or Lady Gaga or any number of queer icons? And to that, I say: Yes. Of course. Before Britney, Madonna, or Beyoncé existed in my little spot in the universe… there was Slipknot.

Growing up in Shepherdsville, Kentucky with a Southern Baptist family during the age of dial up internet, I didn't have gay role models. We weren't even allowed to watch *Will & Grace*. Boys were expected to shoot guns and ride four-wheelers. I'd known I was gay since I was about five. I also knew it was something I shouldn't talk about because, according to my family and my church, that thing about me was bad.

The kids at school in Bullitt County knew I was gay, too, without me even having to say anything. They called me names. They whispered and laughed. One guy named Justin even put me in a chokehold in the hallway between classes once. I passed out.

When I hit puberty, things got really wild. I had all of these feelings pent up inside of me, and in Bullitt County they don't exactly teach men how to express their feelings. I was sad. Incredibly lonely. Disappointed that I was gay because that meant if my family knew, they wouldn't love me. Furious that God knew, and because of that, God didn't love me. I felt caught between being the best little boy in the world and wanting to punch holes in my bedroom walls. I had all of these feelings and nowhere to put them.

And then in 2004, I heard a song that gave me that outlet. A song that unlocked my flair for the dramatic. A song that almost felt like my coming out anthem, even though I wouldn't come out for another four years.

It was "Duality" by Slipknot.

Here was this guy in a Leatherface-looking mask, long hair greased back, screaming about the only way to stop the ache he felt was by pushing his fingers into his eyes. The guitar riffs ate through my angst like chainsaws through flesh.

The emotion! The drama! The aggression! The MASKS! I listened to the song on repeat.

I illegally downloaded their entire discography on Limewire and anxiously awaited the release of their next album. I even made a friend through my love of Slipknot! His name was Corey, and when he stayed the night at my house, we watched MTV2 religiously, just in case they showed the music video, where a bunch of grungy people who looked like us wrecked the absolute shit out of this house where the band hosted a concert.

I related to the masks they wore – the horror of them – probably because I, too, wore a mask. I went to church. I got good grades. I was a leader in the Fellowship of Christian Athletes. But under all of that, I longed to caress the faces of all the boys who threatened to beat the shit out of me. At night I dreamed of getting railed by the entire football team. And then I woke up and went to play rhythm guitar for the church worship band.

I started wearing black T-shirts. I started wearing those jelly bracelets that were all the rage. Studded belts. I was not wearing properly-fitting clothes or making any sort of fashion-forward statements, mind you. But dare I say it… I was beginning to accessorize. To pay attention to my clothing choices. My clothes began to match because black matches everything.

All of my spending money went to Hot Topic. I dyed my hair black and I saved for what seemed like ages so I could buy a Slipknot backpack from Spencer's. I brought my Discman to school and listened to my ripped Slipknot albums. When *Vol. 3: The Subliminal Verses* released I was there at the Wal-Mart, waiting at midnight with Corey for the third shift staff to put the CDs on the shelves. We rode home that night, headbanging and screaming at the top of our lungs with the windows rolled down.

Despite finding a fellow soul who shared my love for horror, heavy music, and masked men

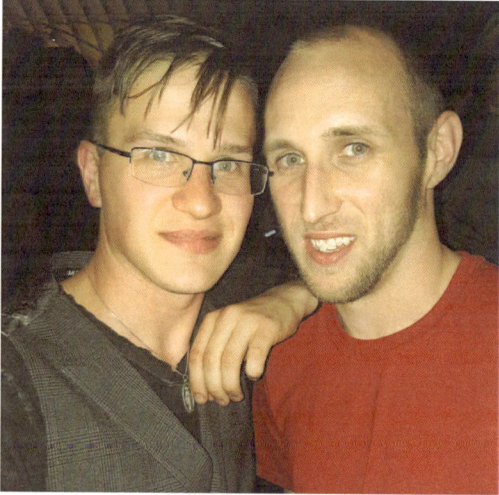

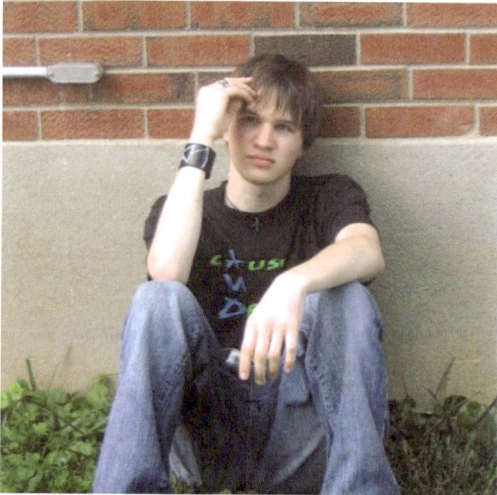

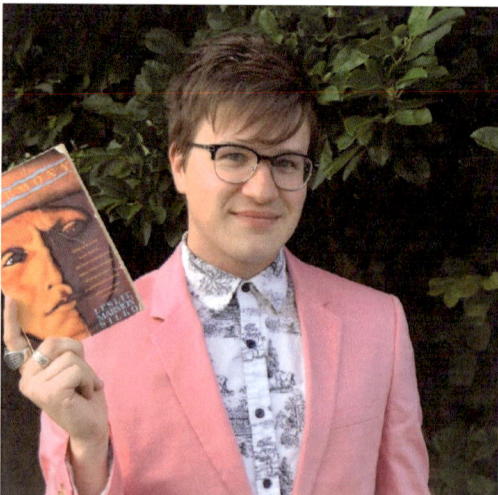

in jumpsuits, I still felt alone. I was still deeply closeted, not even willing to say out loud to myself that I was gay.

A funny thing happened, though. People stopped making fun of me.

After we graduated from high school in 2007, Corey and I fell out of touch like lots of high school friends do. I came out in 2008 and, the last time I'd heard, Corey was dating some girl named Stephanie. But when Slipknot announced they were releasing their album .5:The Gray Chapter, and would be traveling on a tour with a stop in Lexington, who did I call? Corey.

The next thing I knew, we were driving to Lexington together. Even though six years had passed, it felt exactly the same, windows rolled down and growling about pushing our fingers into our eyes. We thrashed our way through that concert, throwing back Miller Lites and sweating through our clothes.

On the way home, we reminisced about concerts of yesteryear, how our families never understood us, and just how sick it was in the music video version of Evanescence's My Immortal when those guitars kicked in. And in all of that, Corey turned to me while I drove us home.

"You remember how I told you I was dating that girl, Stephanie?" he said.

"Yes," I said.

"Well…Stephanie was a 40-year old man named Bob that I met in the locker room of the Downtown YMCA," he said with a devilish grin.

It turns out, after all that time, I wasn't alone. To this day, Corey and I still mosh our way through metal shows together.

And while we love Beyoncé and Lady Gaga and all the rest of them, we still pay homage to our forever queer icons: Slipknot.

photos submitted by Steven Carr   he/him

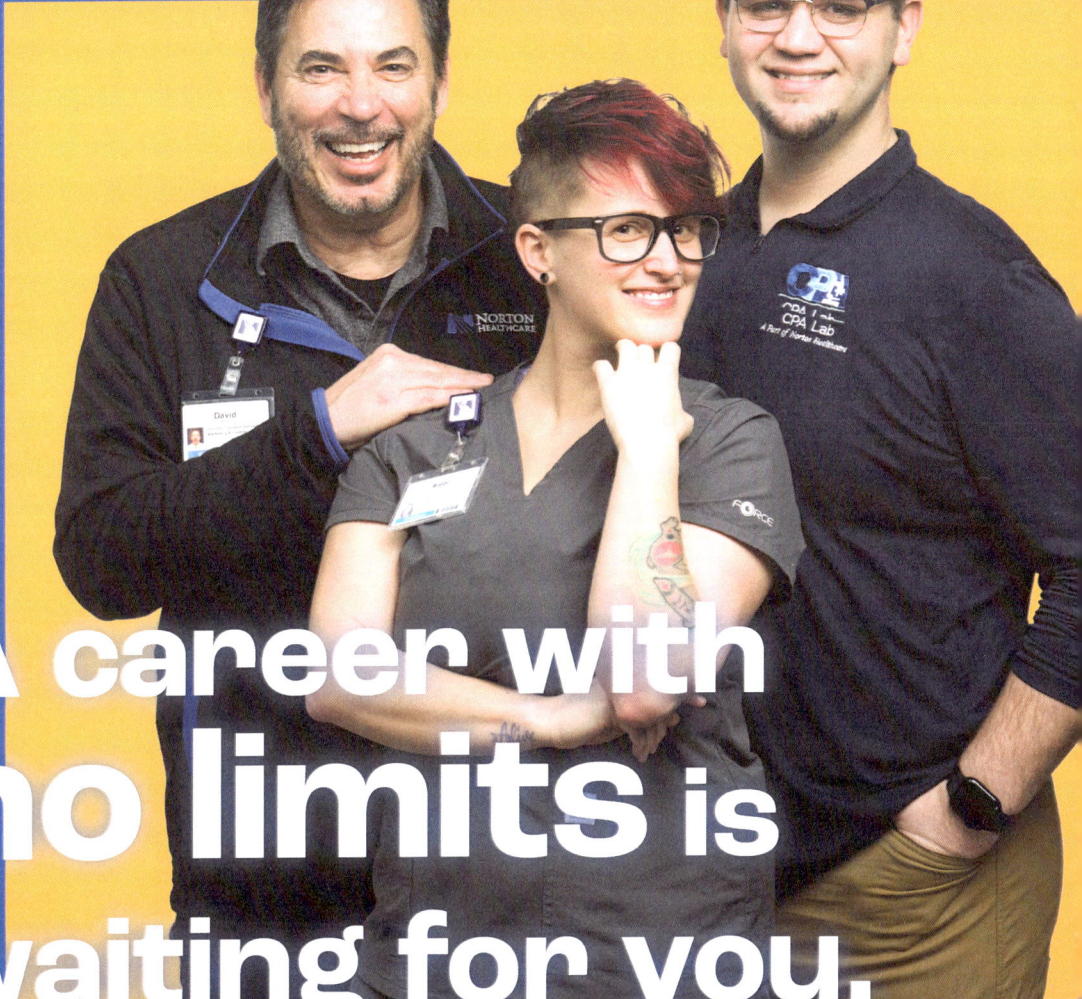

A career with no limits is waiting for you.

Norton Healthcare is unlike any health care system in our region. We're innovators and strategic thinkers. We're researchers, leaders and compassionate caregivers. We're a team — no matter your role or location.

Scan the **QR code** to discover a career with no limits. You can also email **recruitment@nortonhealthcare.org** or call **(800) 833-7975** to speak with a recruiter.

NORTON HEALTHCARE

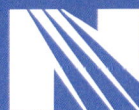

BLACK QUEER AND FREE

Kevin Garner   *he/him   @gearboxlover45*

In our societies, there is an expectation on how we are supposed to act while expressing ourselves as men. This includes how we present ourselves to others. As a Black queer man I have had to "be what it is expected" of me in many situations. Knowing who I am, as well as my worthiness, has been the key to my survival and remains a priceless gift. We are not put here to make others feel comfortable with us. I have felt that as a Black gay man, I was put here to evoke change, teach acceptance and love for all people.

Masculinity is spread throughout our neighborhoods, families, and workplaces. Yet, how we deal with it or "give it a pass" when it rears its ugly head from a toxic perspective is another story. Often the images presented to us in the media can become the norm if we allow it. The images I saw as a young Black boy were the stereotypical images seen in the media — the Marlboro Man and the occasional person of color in a magazine. The only man I had ever seen with a "man bag" was a performance on *Soul Train* with Al Green, now known as the Reverend Al Green. He wore leather shorts, boots to match, and a shoulder bag with a level of masculinity that made me smile and want to go out and get his latest record. I wanted one of those bags because to me it showed me a level of masculinity that I had not seen, but it opened the door to my keen sense of fashion.

Not allowing myself to live in a box is who I am

Not allowing myself to live in a box is who I am today.

today. Luckily, music was very influential to me in those days. Sylvester James, Jr. soon became an essential idol, and to this day, I don't believe there is anyone who can hit those falsetto notes like I did in my bedroom. You see, I was a boy who didn't play with trucks or cars. I was more into shopping with my mother and my record player. This was questioned by some, but not my parents — they knew I was different and that was OK. The arts were my thing. I loved music, movies, fashion, teen magazines and DJ-ing. Music was my salvation! Still is… Prince appeared and my world changed. I never felt that he had a problem embracing his femininity nor masculinity —it appeared to be intertwined within the man. I wanted to be him because criticism did not stop him.

But because I grew up in rural Georgia as a Black boy, I felt that I could not allow my femininity be seen or noticed in public because it was not openly accepted at that time. One of my first experiences of toxic masculinity in my life appeared in my choices for potential love interests. In the 80s, I did not want to be viewed as just a gay man nor was I sure this was how I wanted to identify at the time. I had heard the comments and seen how others who were gay (or believed to be gay) experienced, and I was not there at the time.

I could dish out verbal sparring with the best of them, but I was not going to be OK with the ribbing I would have had to endure so I butched

photo by Sarah Davis   she/her   @sarahkatherinedavisphotography

it up as best I could. To be honest, as a veteran, my masculinity was questioned at times by my peers because I loved loud colors, eyeliner, Benetton, Drakkar Noir and my man crush Pete Burns, the frontman for the English pop band Dead or Alive. There wasn't an abundance of safe spaces at that time. I had survived being a young Black man in the south and I was determined to prosper and survive this.

There are times to this day I feel that masculinity is in the eye of the viewer. Men now can go get their nails done without their masculinity being questioned. Men are now stay-at-home spouses and raise their children. Men are allowing themselves to wear kilts and makeup.

My blueprint to happiness led me down the road of being able to address toxic masculinity situations when and if they presented themselves. Indeed, I made mistakes along the way as you do when you're learning to navigate within your journey to happiness, but I stood up for people who were being ridiculed for simply being themselves – including myself. Becoming openly gay freed me from my unhappiness, and encouraged me to live my life OUTLOUD!

Being Black and queer does have its advantages. We are now role models for others. Being open about how we live, love, and represent is our choice. Breaking down barriers and being unapologetic regarding how we are perceived is now someone else's problem. Our goal now is to not only love each other, but to be out and free. Freedom to be is the ultimate ticket to happiness and I have embraced the journey. I do not allow others to put their sh** on me! Thanks Madonna! There remains work to be done as we fight to build a safer world. Loving yourself and others equals Freedom.

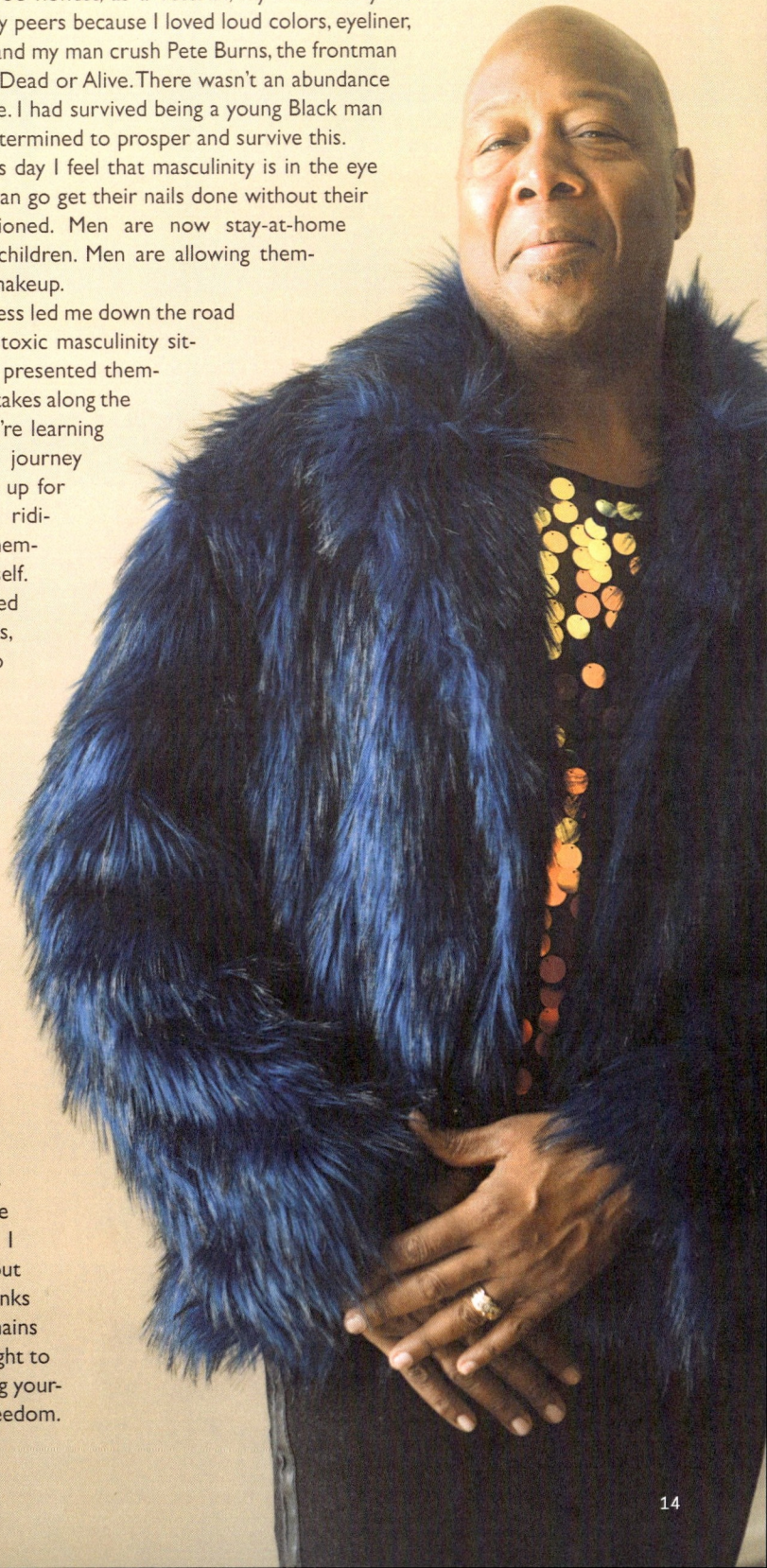

HE PLAYED WITH DOLLS

GROWING UP THROUGH THE MACHISMO EXPERIENCE

Submitted by Luis Ignacio Andrade, Illustration by Andy Mendoza   he/him   @laandymakesart

Luis Ignacio Andrade   *he/him*   *@heplayedwithdolls*

What's that saying— "our parents did the best they could with the tools they were given"? Try telling that to the 12-year-old boy whose mother had just beat him with the Barbie he was playing with, just for playing with it.

"It's gonna be okay; she's only got pliers for that loose screw.
Eventually, she'll get it right."

Or the 6-year-old boy whose dad keeps calling him a "pussy" for crying after punching his tiny little arm as hard as he can. He then spanks him with a belt, because according to him, not being able to sit for a week is an acceptable reason for a boy to cry.

"IKEA gave him the wrong size Allen wrench," you'll tell the boy.
"Don't worry, though; he'll be dead soon."

I was only 10 when my dad accidentally flipped his car into a ditch filled with water and drowned. It didn't take long for the monthly family reunions to stop—a familiar family story. He was the glue that kept the family together, they'd say. Aunts stopped talking to aunts; uncles were no longer forced to speak to other uncles by the aunts; and cousins lost touch. Birthdays and family events such as weddings or quinceañeras were mandatory — otherwise, as we got older, we were allowed to choose which family members we wanted to see. Deciding who to visit on long weekends wasn't hard for me. I could visit the aunt who never smiled and whose husband shamed or hit his sons every time they missed a pass during touch football.

"Ram into him!" He'd order my cousin, asshole Junior. "Use your fucking elbow! Don't be a faggot!"

"Tío, this is touch-football," I'd remind him.

"Go play with the other girls," he'd say back.

Or, I could choose Uncle Manny, the exiled uncle whose wife got into a physical altercation with the aunt who never smiled.

"Let's go play in my room," my cousin Monica suggested as soon as we walked in the front door the weekend after my 13th birthday. We ran to her room, locked the door behind us, and gathered all her Barbies and their clothes.

"My Barbie is going to wear boots with her dress," I said as I held one pink lace-up knee-high boot and hunted for the other. "Got it!"

As I combed Barbie's hair, the story I gave her began to bring her to life. The more life I gave Barbie, the safer I felt in the world I was creating for her—for us. I was still feeling on edge from the last time I had gotten caught playing with dolls.

"Cual quierres? Which one do you want? The pink one?" My mother yelled as she threw my sister's dresses at me. "You're a boy! Boys don't play with dolls! You want me to send you to school in this one!" Mommy Dearest continued, smacking me across the face with another dress as my sister watched, hiding behind a pillow. Crying.

"No!" I begged.

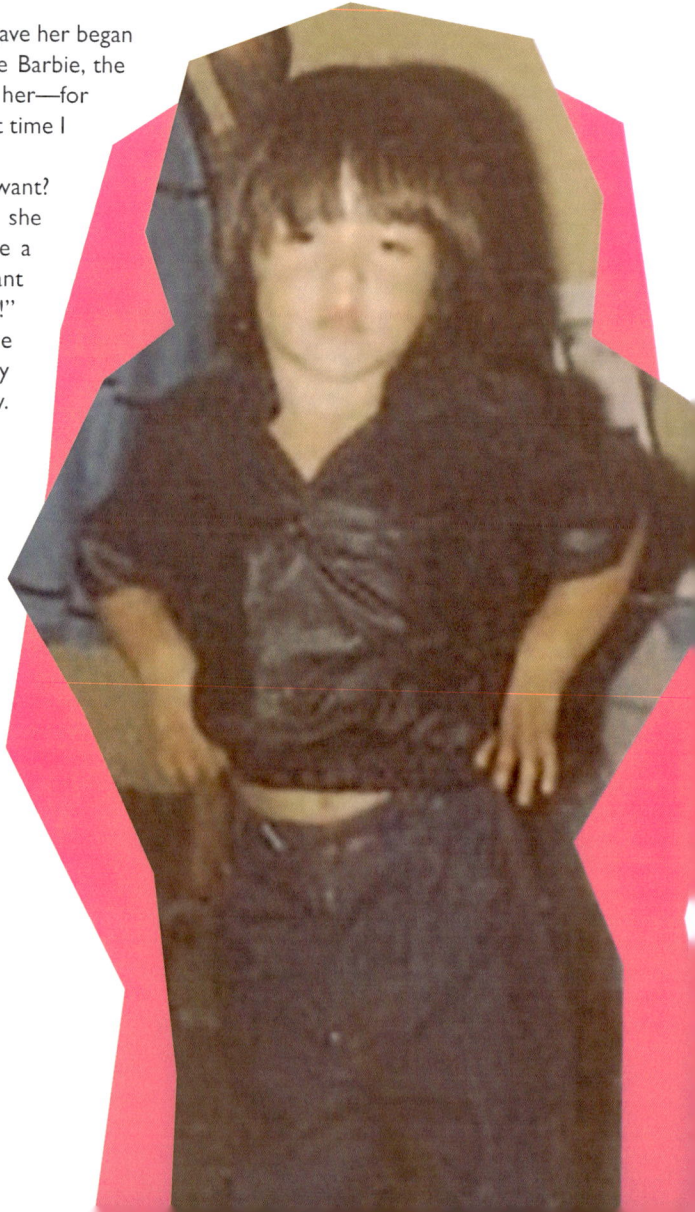

"HE SMILED AT ME, CONFIRMING WHAT MONICA HAD ASSURED. THAT WITH THEM, I WAS SAFE."

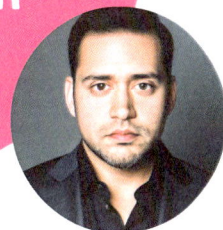

She thought she could scare the femininity out of me by threatening embarrassment. What she didn't realize was that sending me to school in a dress would end me. The boys at school were beating me up. Teasing me for having a soft voice and hanging around with girls. I couldn't imagine what would happen to me if I showed up in a dress.

"She's a model. And Ken's an actor," I said. "But he cheated on Barbie with a co-star, Christie, so now my Barbie will murder them." My stories always ended with someone getting murdered, usually being telenovela-slapped off a chest of drawers imagined as the Empire State Building.

"What do you think about her hair? She just got out of the salon," Monica said, twirling her Barbie displaying every angle of her off-center ponytail.

"It's beautiful," I lied. "What do you think about…" Fear instantly flooded my body. We forgot to lock the door. I threw the Barbie, but it was already too late. Uncle Manny walked in and made the face of someone accidentally walking into an occupied dressing room. My heart pounded against my chest. I was sure he would yell at me and forbid me to come over again. Who wouldn't? Only weird boys play with toys meant for girls.

He slowly entered the room, closed the door behind him, and locked it. I closed my eyes, waiting for my punishment. I felt him walk past me, opened my eyes, and saw him pick up the Barbie I had thrown across the room, now, lying face down on the floor, missing a boot. He handed her to me. He sat on the floor, picked up a brush, and the recently murdered Christie. As he began to brush her hair, he asked me in his soft voice, "What's your Barbie going to wear to the party tonight, Nachito?"

I looked over at Monica. "He plays with us all the time," she said, assuring me it was okay. I watched while Uncle Manny played with Christie—a big, tall man with a soft voice brushing a doll's hair. He smiled at me, confirming what Monica had assured. That with them, I was safe.

When we finally learn to accept that our parents did their best with the tools they were given by God or the Universe, their parents or Grandparents, or even YouTube, it's easier to move through the shame. I think that's true for everyone.

The wrong tools, I imagine, are dumped into our own unorganized toolboxes in the form of shame, rejection, and fear that we then have to dig through or discard as we experience our own lives. Mom, before the screw was stripped too far, eventually figured out the proper tool to use. I like to think that somewhere along the way, had he survived the accident, my dad would have been given that Allen wrench.

At Uncle Manny's funeral, I told Monica that her dad was the first person in my life that made me feel accepted and that I belonged.

"How did he do that?" she asked.

I smiled, held her hand, and said, "he played with dolls."

TRANS FELICITY

DELTA 400   PROFESSIONAL

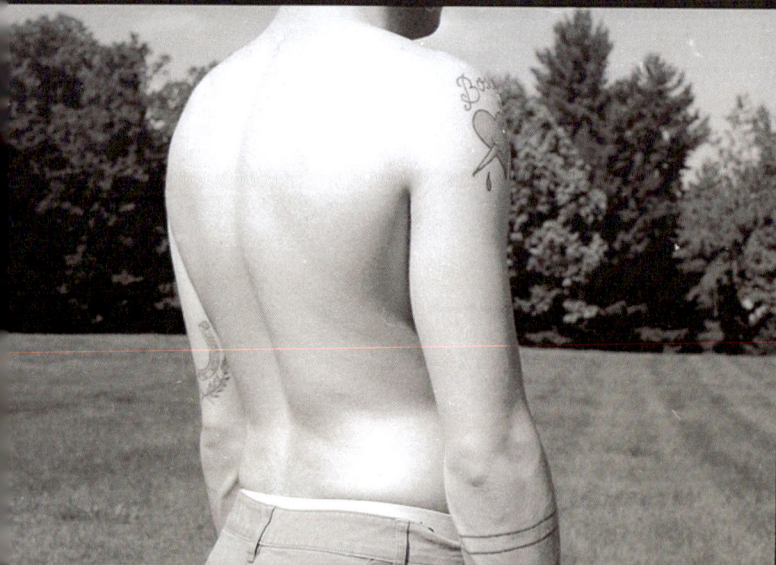

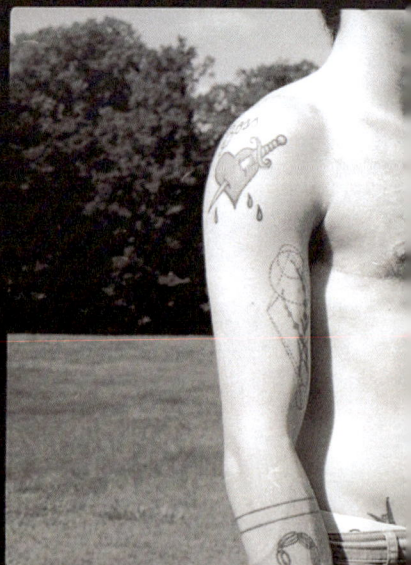

12 ►12A 13

Shooting film since 2012, Lane Levitch finally steps in front of his own camera. Before, he didn't like seeing how the world perceived him. His face so permanent on negative strips. After receiving a gender affirming surgery in August 2022, Lane started documenting his healing process and stepping into his confidence. He was taking digital photographs until the passing of his life-long friend, Henry Berg-Brousseau, when he switched to film. The digital photos felt too casual for a surgery that's so life changing. He now embraces the permanence of film.

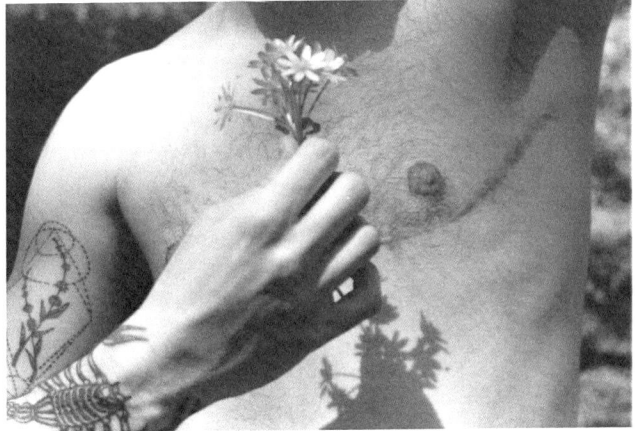

Lane Levitch *he/him* *@lnlvtch*

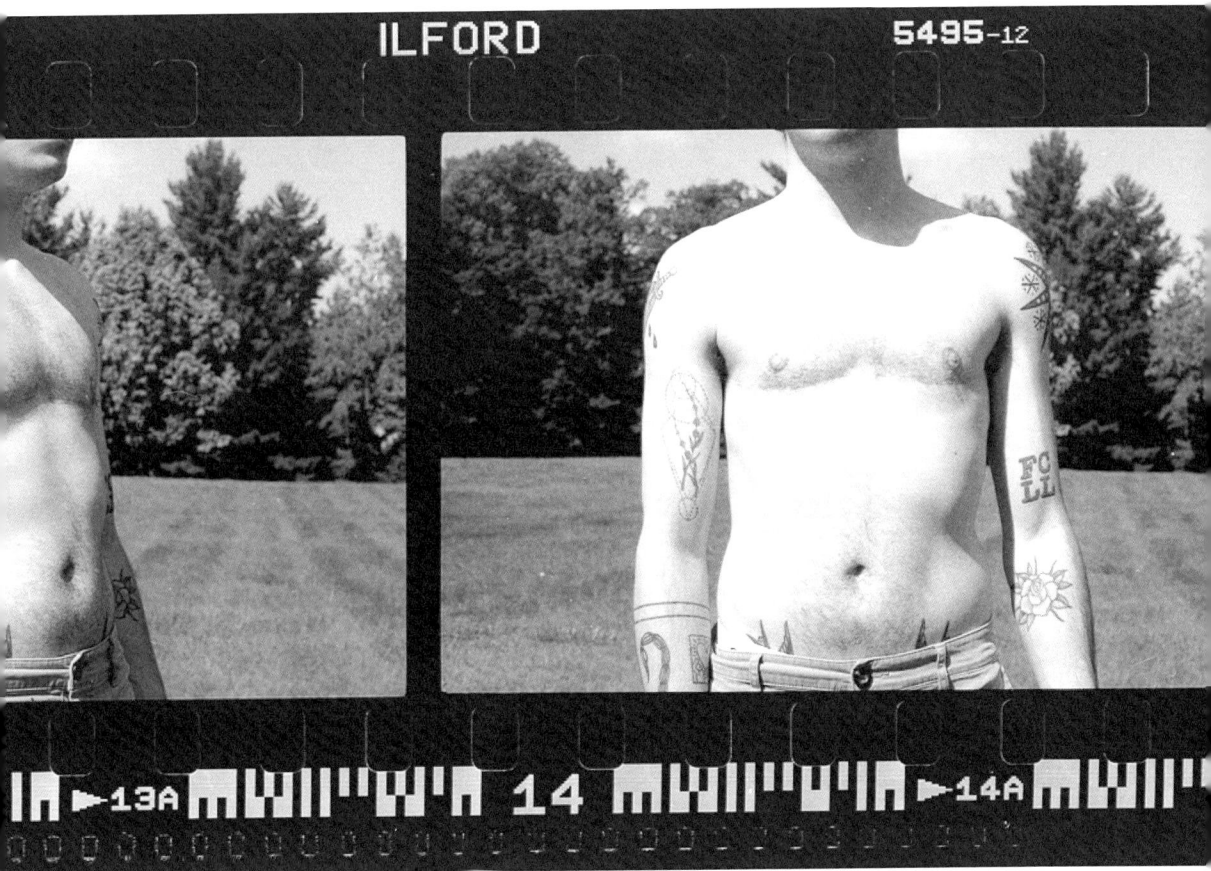

ILFORD 5495-12

13A 14 14A

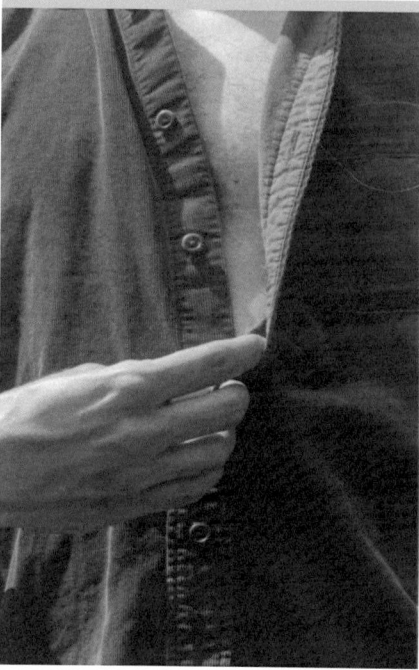

Trans Felicity is a celebration of transgender joy and self respect. Taking self portraits in nature, Lane gets to do something he always dreamed of: Being shirtless with the sun touching his skin.

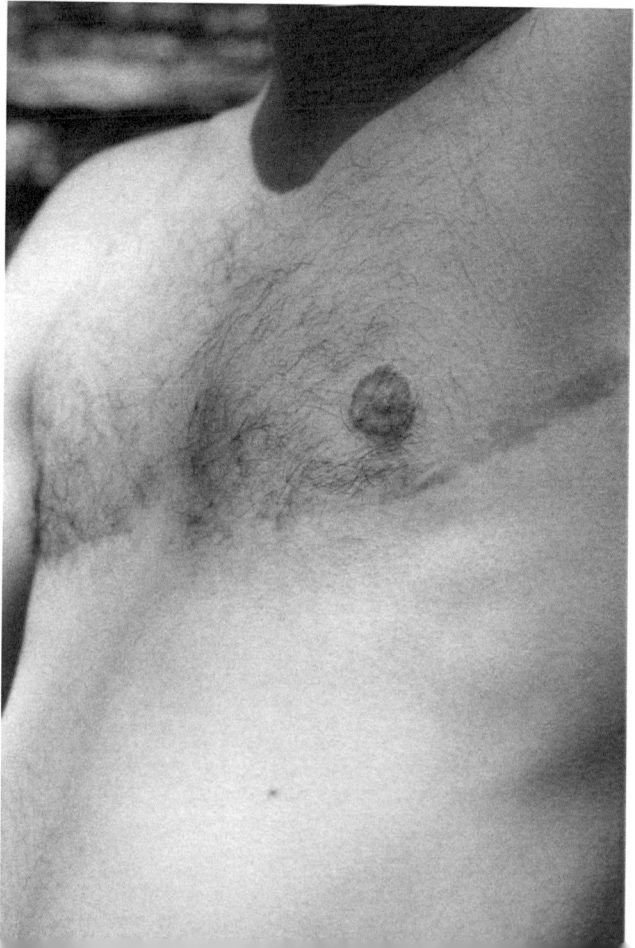

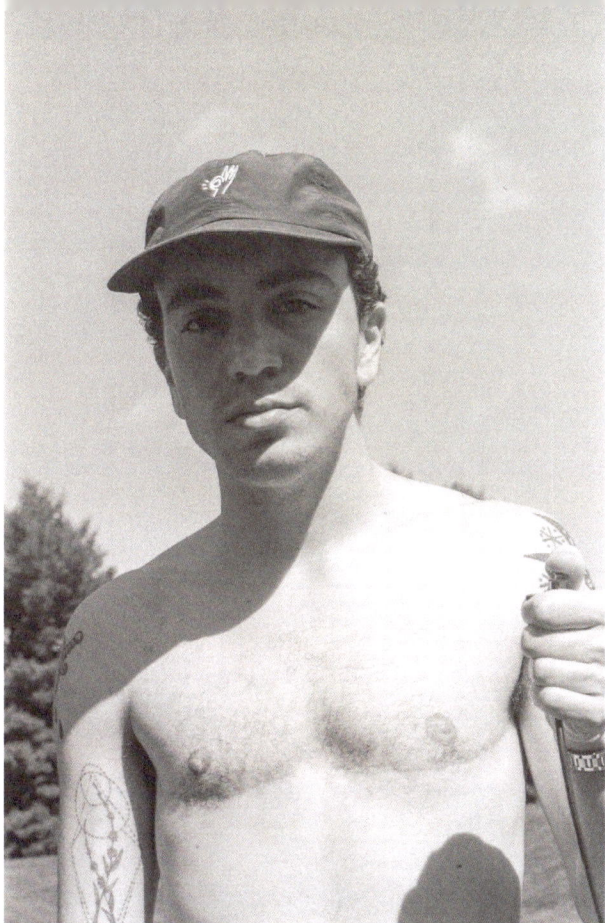

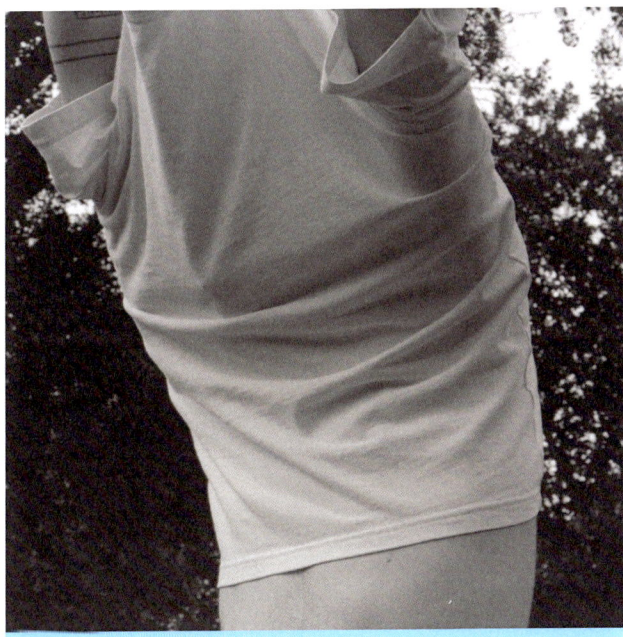

Trans Felicity is meant to stand still in time, to bottle up the happiness from the year following surgery. To be a reminder for Lane that he has come a long way in his gender journey, but also as a reminder to trans youth that it does, in fact, get better.

LAVENDER COUNTRY

"A VIBE THAT'S WORTH THE DRIVE"

Austyn Gaffney she/her @austyngaffney

At Little Mount Lavender, about a mile off the outlet mall exit in Simpsonville, Kentucky, both owners, both named Jason, own what they say is the largest year-round lavender store on the Eastern seaboard.

Both Jasons are also in love: Jason Woodlief married Jason Walker, who subsequently became Walker-Woodlief, in 2014, with an officiant and a witness in New York City, a year before the Supreme Court legalized same-sex marriage. Three years later, the couple bought property in Taylorsville, moved their horses and their dog Hank out of South Carolina, where Woodlief grew up, and started planting what would become ten thousand plants of Lavandula intermedia Phenomenal, a French lavender hybrid.

"Neither of us knew anything about lavender," said Walker-Woodlief, over coffee and sweet tea in the store's cafe. But they started researching a long-term, alternative crop. At first they just sold directly from their fields, tying the lavender into bundles and hanging them from their barn ceiling along tobacco sticks. But then, he said, "It got out of control."

"I made him rent the store before the lavender was even blooming yet," said Woodlief. The store was 300-square-feet in Shelbyville.

Quickly outgrowing the space, they expanded into a downtown storefront over tenfold the size of their original shop, adding a bakery (Walker-Woodlief is a trained pastry chef) and a manufacturing hub for their mind-numbing supply of lavender merch. They produced lotions, soaps, candles, teas, diffusers, and then packaged it all together into gift sets.

"Loyalty was key," said Woodlief of their customers. His husband, wearing trademark overalls, filmed videos of the farm and the lavender to engage with them. "They became committed to us because we were so involved."

Woodlief and Walker-Woodlief chose lavender because it was a perennial, it was hardy, and it had an ever-expanding array of uses. Lavender has been used for its medical properties since the middle ages — with

Photos were submitted by Little Mount Lavender, taken by Anthony Munger

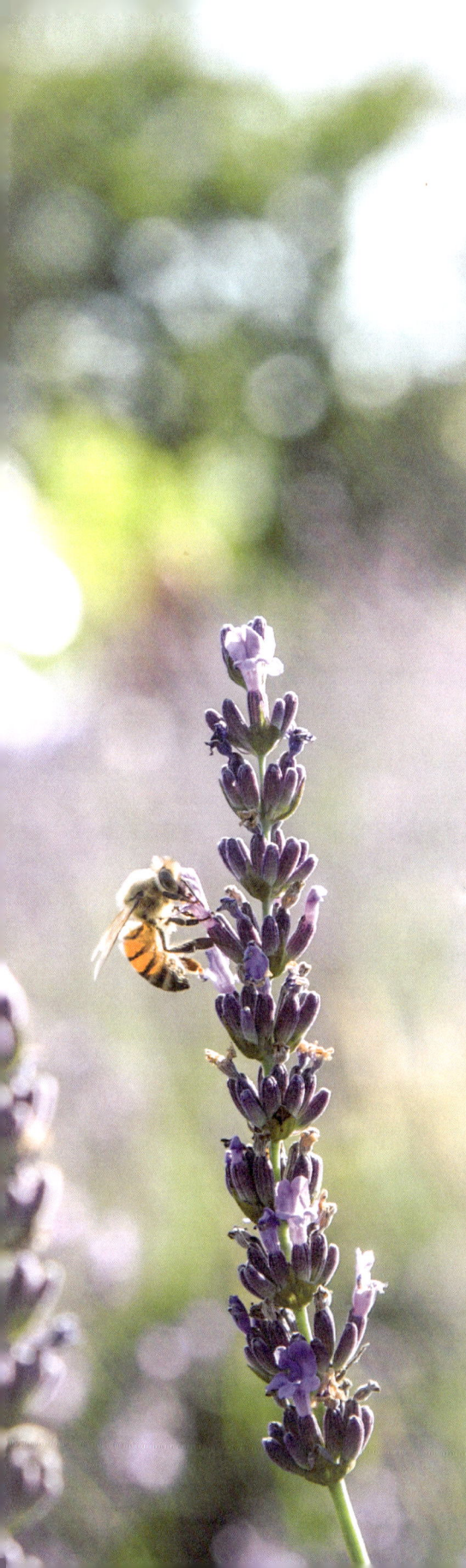

its antibacterial, antifungal, and antimicrobial properties, lavender is a common ingredient in herbal medicines, along with cosmetics, food, and aromatherapy.

With all the merchandising potential, their nascent business stretched further. In 2021, they moved the shop about seven miles west on Shelbyville Road and into the Old Stone Inn, an 1811 renovated tavern that takes the mantle as the oldest stone residence in Shelby County.

Before they took it over, the building, most recently a restaurant, was abandoned like in an apocalypse movie. Food soured in the kitchen. Squirrels left nuts on the staircases. The spouses used 75 gallons of white paint to rehab the space, hired ten associates, and turned the upstairs rooms into production. They'd previously visited lavender shops in California, and Woodlief thought, "We can do as good or better," than those shops.

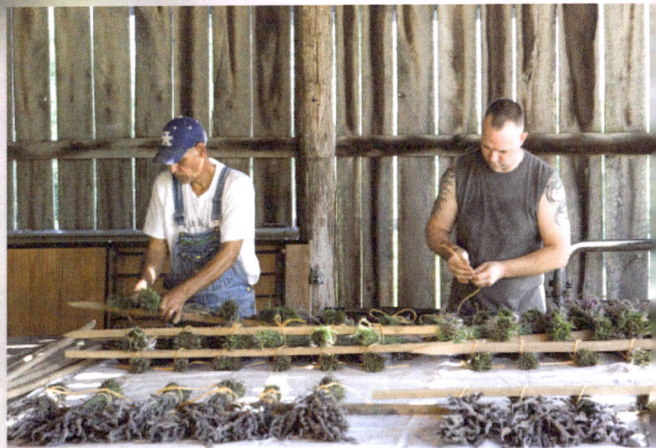

Now, with faux-crystal chandeliers, clean walls, and gleaming wood floors, Walker said the vibe of the shop was "French glitter." Woodlief, who got his start at Wal-Mart and Amazon, continued expanding the store as he discovered more products. Now, the Old Stone Inn, with its astronomical amount of lavender and lavender-adjacent products, is sort of like a Buc-ee's, but more purple and more gay (and closer to Louisville than Lexington). In a commercial, Walker-Woodlief calls his store, "A vibe that's worth the drive."

That vibe appears the minute I walk through the shop's front door where a 40-foot lavender carpet unrolls. Along the hallway are bamboo charcoal toothbrushes, bamboo soap dishes, all-natural hand towels, wool dryer balls, and organic bath bombs. Through a doorway, there is an entire wall of soy candles and another of eco-friendly dishcloths. There are long-stemmed matches with lilac tips, lavender sachets, bundles of dried lavender, soft fleece lavender throws, and lavender silicone pot lids. In another of the shop's five rooms, there are throw pillows, oven mitts, aprons, and mugs. There are wheat straw dining sets, car cup holder coasters and car cup holder coaster sets. There are wooden bow ties and there are shelves upon shelves of crystals. Some crystals advertise forgiveness while others are "all about opening your Heart and mind to your True Self!"

At the back, there is a bakery, and in the bakery are fresh-baked French baguettes, lavender creme brulee and lavender lemon cake, lavender dark chocolate cookies and lavender coconut cookies. There is lavender-infused olive oil, lavender-infused balsamic vinegar, and lavender-based seasoning mixes.

Outside the cafe, where comfort food like soup, pasta, and shepherd's pie is served, are twelve rows of lavender in a sloping lawn bordering the roadside. Here, school groups visit, as do local churches and community groups. Beyond their wares, another vibe is different in Simpsonville than in Shelbyville, says the husbands. In Shelbyville, four months after opening, they were interviewed for an article in the town's local paper, The Sentinel-News. Before it ran, the paper mentioned it would leave out the detail that Woodlief and Walker-Woodlief were married.

"Then don't print the story," Walker-Woodlief told them. While he said he felt the editor was trying to be sensitive to both his readership and their business, Walker-Woodlief said that if their identity bothered a potential customer, "They were probably not our customer." The reporter added their marriage back into the story, and came to the store in person to apologize.

The couple said their sexuality never seemed to be a problem in either town, but since opening, the shop has typically been a place for women to come meet friends, says Woodlief. Around 11a.m., two women come giggling into the cafe, one in a light purple cardigan, and they order cocktails in lavender hues. While they sit chatting in the corner of the cafe, Walker-Woodlief notes that this is their typical customer — female and over 40. But lately, they've noticed more women bringing their husbands and boyfriends.

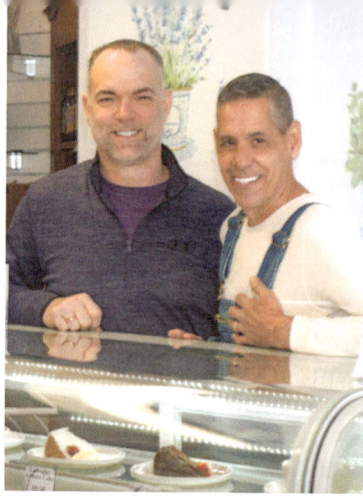

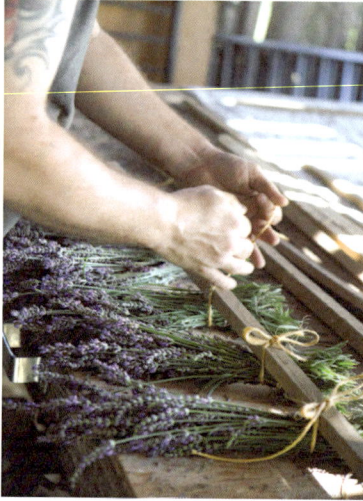

"Self-care is more normalized, and it's trendier for men to take care of themselves," says Walker-Woodlief. So their product line is moving towards wellness. They experiment at home with new ideas before selling items in the store. Right now, they're beta testing face masks and snail mucin, a moisturizer made from the tiny slime trails of tiny snails. Their shop, he adds, and how the couple interacts with their community, is part of breaking the hard habit of toxic masculinity.

After the coffee, back in my car, I couldn't help but play the title track of the 1973 album Lavender Country, what's widely considered the first openly gay country album. As I pulled out of the parking lot, on the title track, singer-songwriter Patrick Haggerty crooned,

"There's nothing left but holes
In your weary sexist roles...
You all come out, come out, my dears
To Lavender Country"

So, come out: Little Mount Lavender is open Monday through Saturday from 10am-6pm, with lunch served in the cafe from 10am-4pm.

Little Mount Lavender 6905 Shelbyville Rd, Simpsonville, KY

THE DADDY SISTERS
"BEAST WITH TWO BACKS"

SPRING 2024

sona BLAST!

✨ **Business support that meets you where you are!** ✨

Inclusive and training-focused business support

Website Design | Branding Design
Graphic Design | Marketing Support

Alight Agency is Queer, Appalachian, and Woman Owned,
ready to help you run your business with confidence and joy. ✨

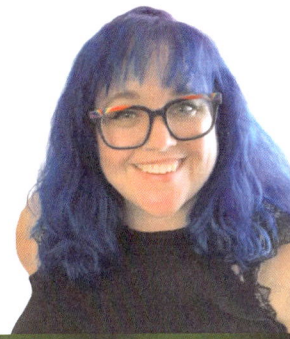

AlightAgency.com | @AlightAgency | (859) 351-3542

Quality, Integrity & Knowledge
Matter!

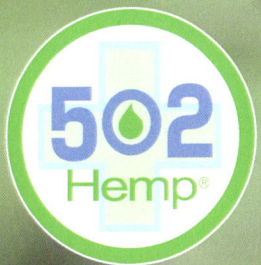

Your Cannabis Connection.

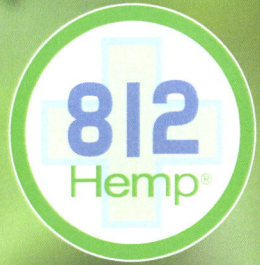

502 Hemp Wellness Center
201 Moser Rd., Suite B
Louisville, KY
502.654.7100
502hemp.com

812 Hemp
319 E. Lewis and Clark Pkwy.
Clarksville, IN
812.913.0045
812hemp.com

Save 10% online.

Code: Welcome10

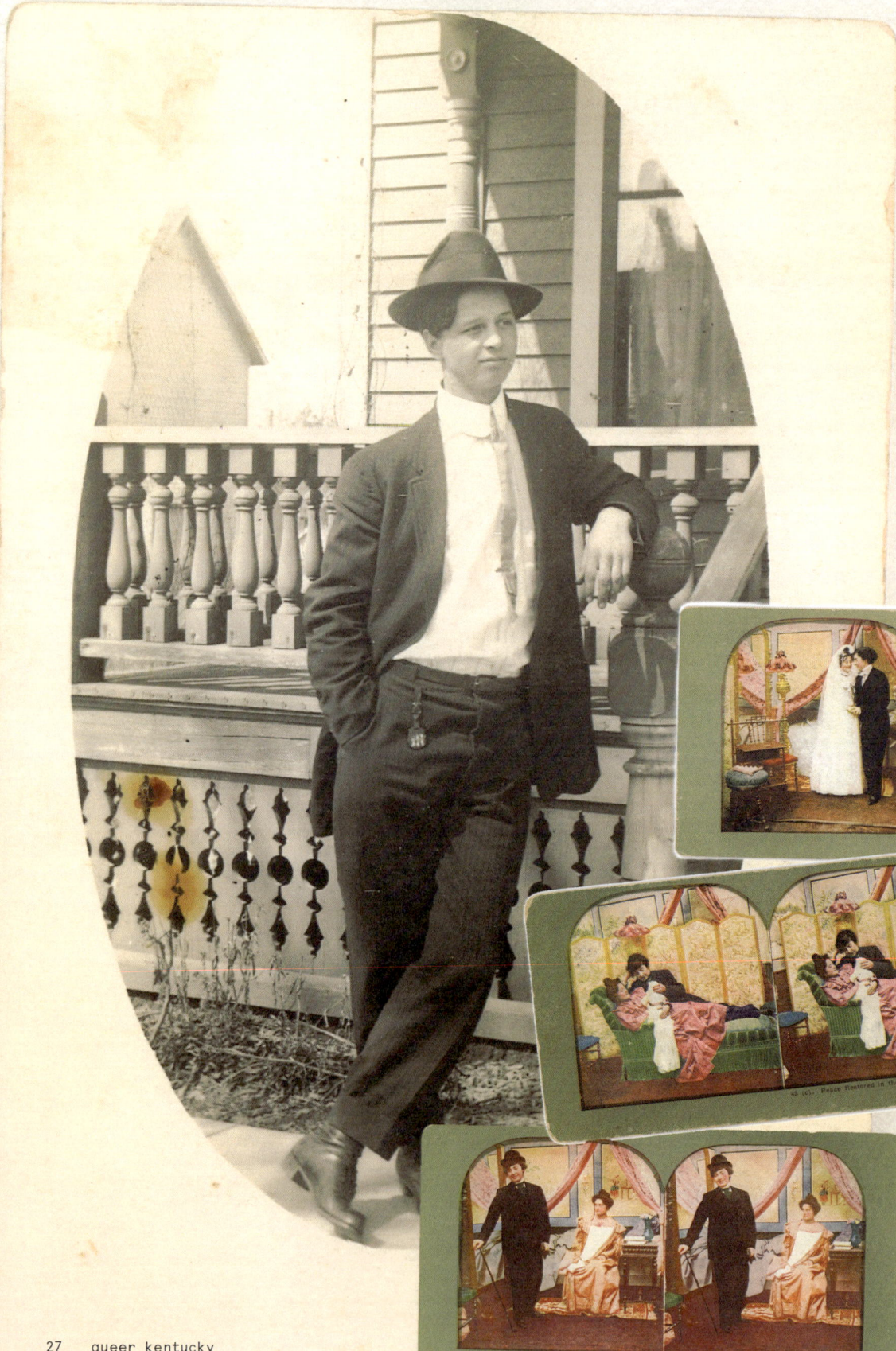
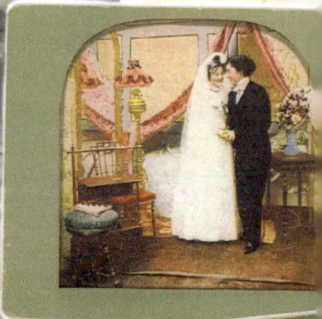
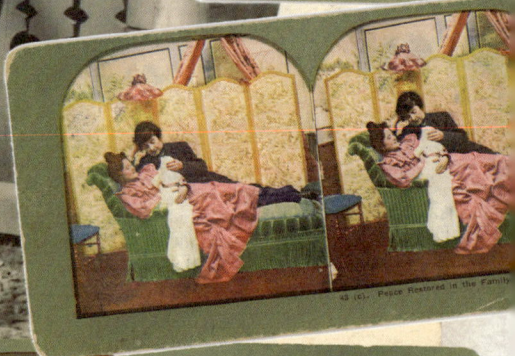
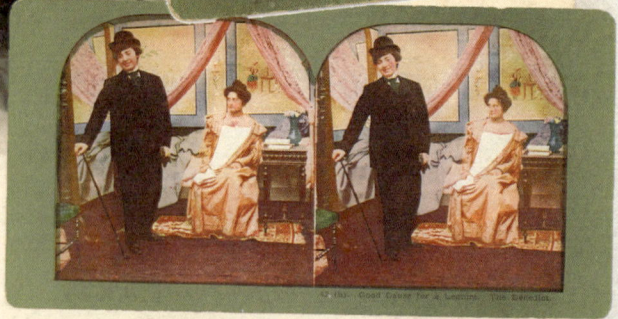

A Brief Butch History

Faulkner Morgan Historical Archive
@faulknermorganarchive

The term "butch," commonly associated with LGBTQ+ women, originated from a robust lesbian subculture in the mid-1900s. While its cultural meaning has since shifted and is now widely used among many different genders and sexualities, it is still predominantly used to describe masculine-presenting women. In our collections at Faulkner Morgan Archive, we have a wide range of items showcasing a deep history of butch women from long before the term even came to be used as a queer marker.

Clothing has often served as a central aspect of one's gender expression, particularly within the LGBTQ+ community. Take one of our favorite photos in the archive, for instance. While we do not know the exact date, location, or subjects of the image, we are still able to explore a queer reading of what we see. The women in these photos are wearing loose-fitting, masculine clothing. We can even see the cuffs are rolled up (pretty substantially, we might add) as this style of clothing was not made to fit women at that time. There also seems to be an immense joy and confidence radiating from their faces.

How do we know that images we have collected are queer though? We have no idea who these items originally belonged to or who is depicted, but we do know how they were acquired in Kentucky. We have many postcards and photographs from flea markets, yard sales, and antique stores, from donors across the state. One of these donors described how he was always looking for "sissy men" and "manly women" and that the photographs had to show, in this collector's estimation, "that look, somewhere in the eyes." Many of the photographs that we have collected display elements of cross-dressing or close, intimate contact. All the photographs are anonymous, but for their collectors, they represent an early LGBTQ+ presence in this state.

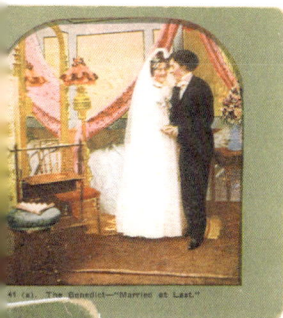

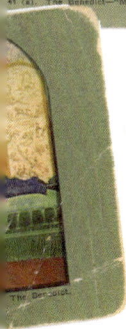

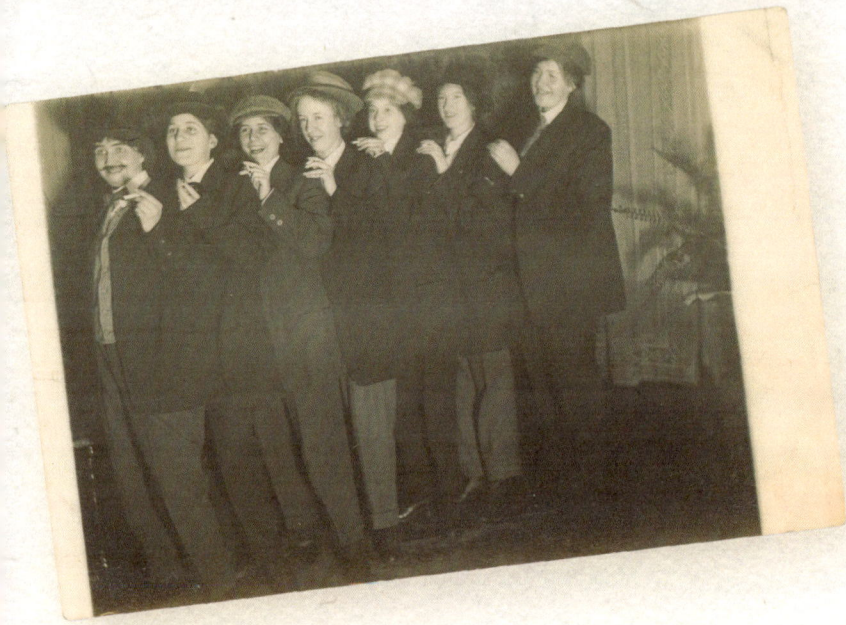

they exclaimed that "'Mr. Bark' Was A Woman." Prior to their death, Bark had shared with a neighbor that, as it was more difficult for women to make a living for themselves at that time, living as a man more easily allowed them to survive. While this story raises complex questions about our understanding of gender identity in the early 20th century, it is clear that dressing masculine was Bark's way of survival.

As time has progressed, we begin to see a less binary understanding of gender and sexuality. Faulkner Morgan Archive, in our mission to save and share Kentucky's LGBTQ history, also records queer Kentucky now, as it is

Found at a flea market in Georgetown, these stereoscopic cards play quite openly with same-sex desire, featuring two women getting married. Even in this same-sex marriage, though, one of the women is clearly dressed more masculine or butch. The two women then go on to even have a baby. The one in masculine dress asks "I wonder where the baby got her blue eyes?" For some, this could just be a humorous, slightly-edgy parlor joke. But if you're a woman who loves women living in Kentucky around the year 1900, these cards could be a revelation—that other forms of love and family can exist.

Oftentimes, masculine clothing and other non-femme appearances acted as visual cues to subtly (or not so subtly) indicate queerness to others. They could also potentially signify more than simple masculine dress, but also a masculine identity. At the time, these simple differences of dress were seen as deviant and abnormal. One article that we've found, published in 1903, unveils how a community reacted to someone wearing clothing that didn't match their assigned sex at birth.

Aaron Bark of Muhlenberg County was outed after their death as a "woman… dressed in men's clothes." When this was discovered by the community,

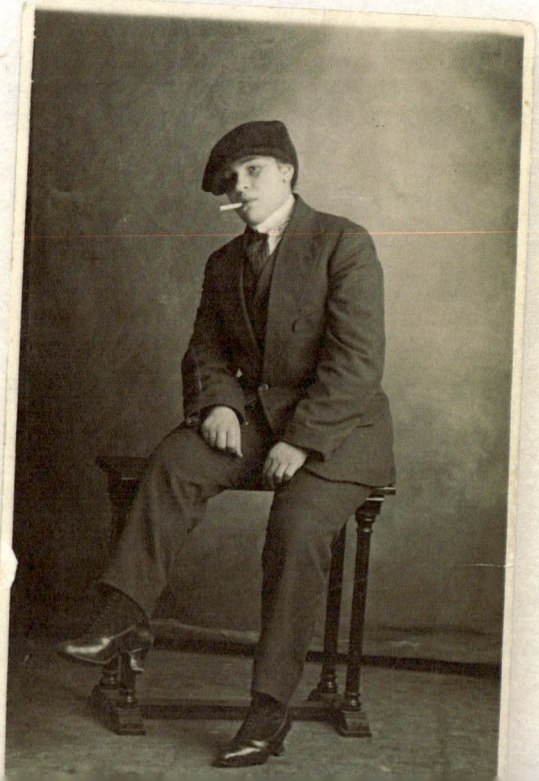

happening. *Ian Smoking* by Louisville-based artist Casie Lewis is a perfect example. Through their bold images, Lewis captures the complexity and frivolity of their circle of trans and genderqueer friends in Kentucky. These photos, in particular, play with butchness and the gender ambiguity that surrounds butchness. Masculinity is emphasized in this genderqueer imagery.

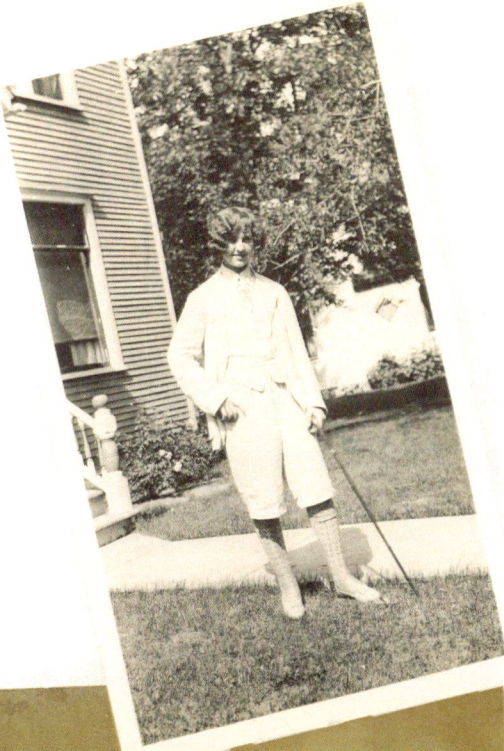

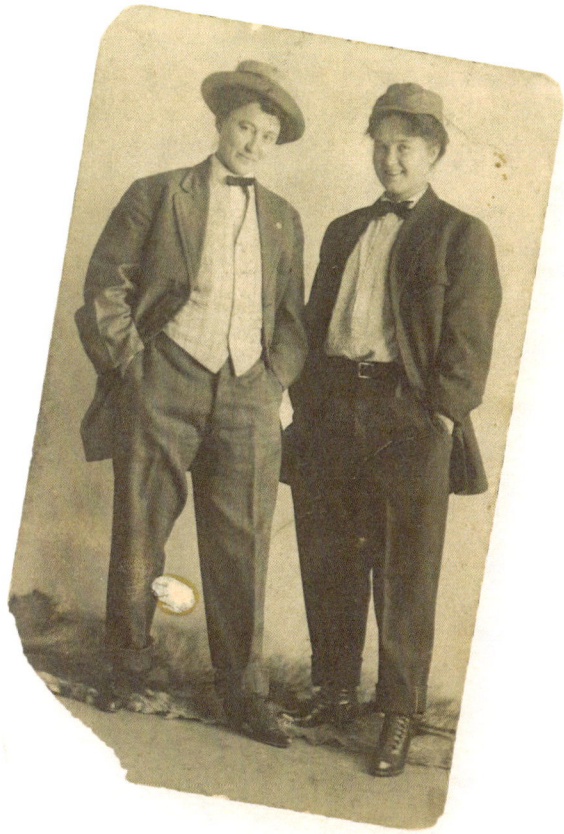

The Faulkner Morgan Archive works to shed light on the deep historical roots of the LGBTQ+ community in Kentucky. Through archived photos such as these, the significance of representing varied gender expression becomes evident. By exploring this brief, yet rich, butch history, we share stories that not only acknowledge struggles and triumphs but also to foster a profound sense of belonging.

The Faulkner Morgan Archive is a grassroots community archive with a mission to share Kentucky's LGBTQ history. Our collections span 200 years of history, representing individuals, events, and institutions across Kentucky's diverse LGBTQ spectrum, creating a rich resource for activists, scholars, artists, museums, and the curious. We believe sharing our history can change our future. You can find us online at FaulknerMorgan.org or on Facebook and Instagram @FaulknerMorganArchive.

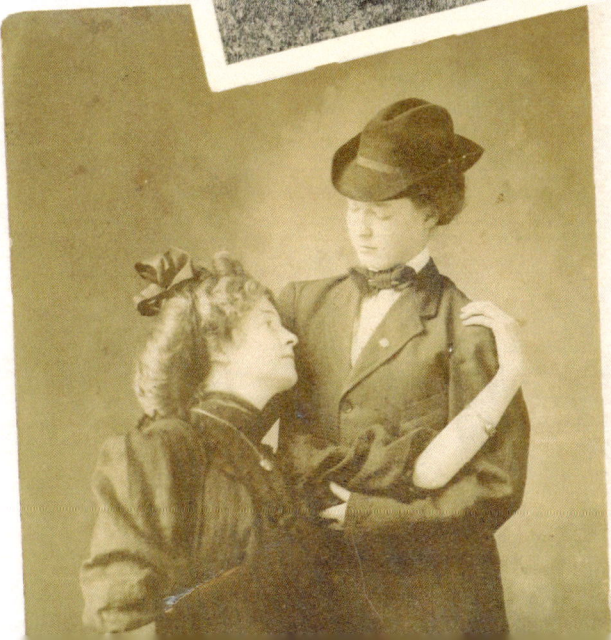

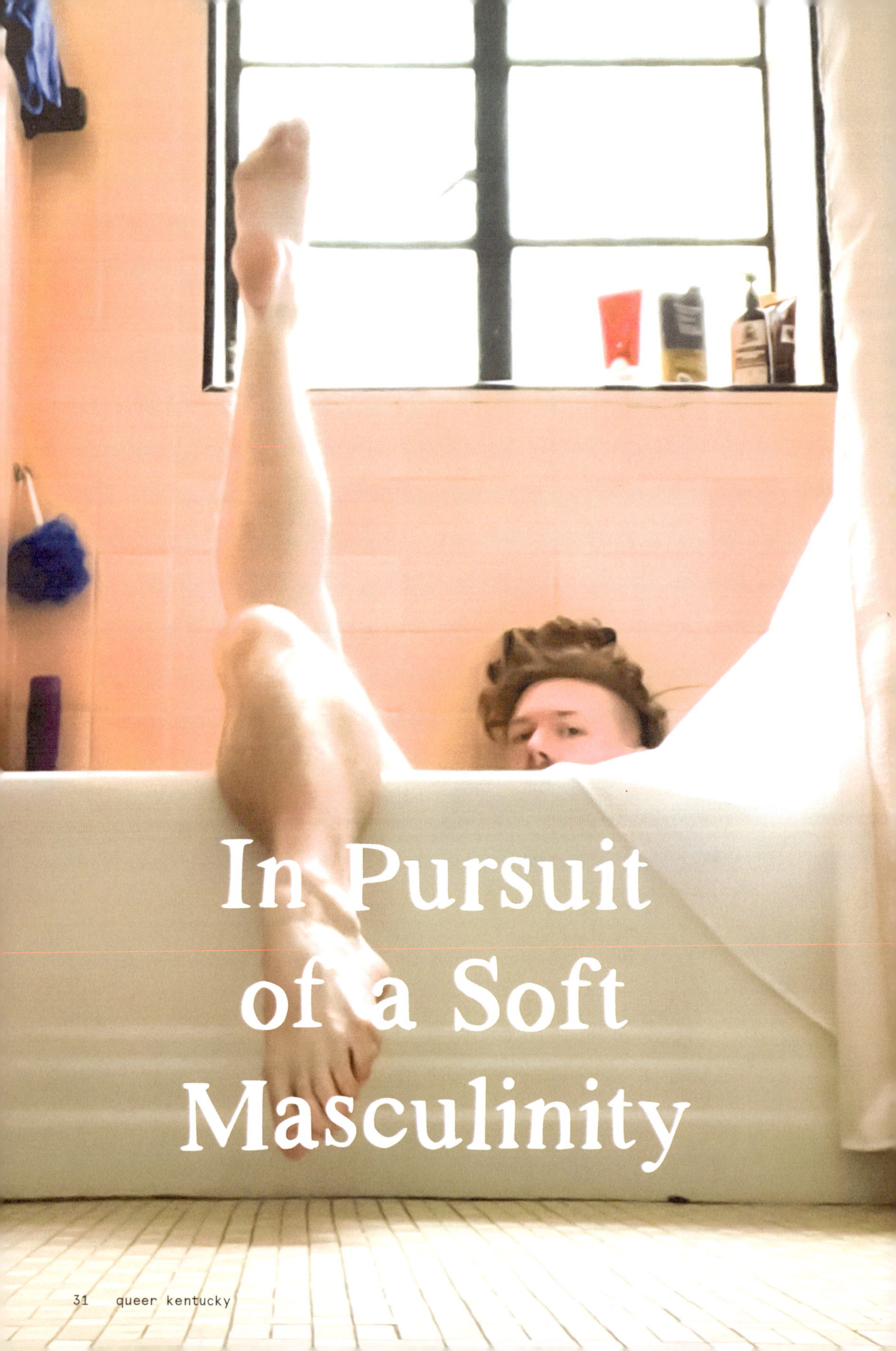

In Pursuit of a Soft Masculinity

A He/They's Tell-All

Joshua Brown *he/they* *@meth.borrison*

I grew up homeschooled in an Evangelical household — a notoriously supportive environment for a deeply queer future-artist. While my parents were and continue to be very supportive, the ideology I was exposed to was less so. I also grew up in the mid-'90s, and this meant my understanding of binary gender was dictated by the McDonald's drive-through: Hot Wheels for boys, Barbie for girls. As a child, having two very powerful deities (Jesus and Ronald McDonald) ascribe to rigid pink-and-blue gender divisions was a major source of stress. This stress wasn't as much due to my desire to transgress these boundaries, but a frustration that they existed at all.

I was never comfortable being categorized, but there was something particularly inescapable about the labels "boy" and "man." From bathrooms, to department stores, to toys, games, and cartoons, everything seemed to have a binary spin to it. As a kid, I always felt confronted by the color blue, as if it were always saying "this is for you, you should like this!" It rarely was, and I rarely did. Instead, the kinds of toys and media I genuinely enjoyed were often locked behind what I felt was a pink-hued electric fence. As I got older, this division widened to include not only media, but creative interests, sports, and community.

I have a vivid memory of asking my mother if I could start gymnastics classes when we lived in South Florida, and her response was "that's a girl's sport." This response was informed by her own experience as a moderately-ok young gymnast, surrounded by hyperactive girls in lycra handled by strong and supportive male coaches. But when I eventually watched the Olympics for the first time and saw that team of muscled short kings winning gold for their floor routines, I felt a bit betrayed. My fear was never being the only boy in a group of girls; it was always being one boy in a sea of others.

Whether I was being shunted into gendered Bible study groups, mocked for enjoying *Sailor Moon* and *Cardcaptor Sakura*, or given different chores than my sister, I always felt indignant when someone used gender as justification for curating my behavior. Even small comments like "men stand up straight and tall" or "boys are stronger" would spark my fury. My most egregious faux pas happened when I joined a Lego robotics group at age ten. All the boys went around and introduced themselves with their name and favorite superhero, and I, in a dazzling show of social candor, said "my name is Josh Brown, and I hate them all."

All of this to say, I was not only resistant to traditional masculinity, I was terrible at it. So terrible, in fact, that by the time I was a sophomore in high school with a real-life girlfriend, these tensions that had been bubbling would quickly boil over.

At 15-years-old, deviations from the gender binary would amount less to silly social faux pas and more to fundamental questions of identity. Rather than the simple answer that I was a flaming homosexual, my logic held that I was still straight, just sensitive. In some ways, this was a positive delusion. I convinced myself that straight men could resist the stereotypes foisted on them and be complex individuals — and I was one of them. I was "straight," yet I had meaningful friendships with women; I loved poetry and theatre; I didn't care about sports or superheroes or cars; I loved '80s pop divas, etc. This sensitive heterosexuality was comfortable for my indoctrinated mind for the dual purposes of staving off the certain damnation I would suffer as a homo and allowing me to express my genuine interests free of judgment. After all, the more traditionally masculine one appears and acts, the more endearing transgressions of the gender binary become.

As my girlfriend and I shared our signature single, closed-lip kiss for the tenth time with no risk of going further, I was proud of my sensitive masculinity. I was kind and cute and silly and loved playing the oboe, and that felt transgressive in its own special way. Even as that relationship fell apart and I embraced my sexuality in college, the allure of a softer masculinity never left me. Queer men, shockingly, are still men, and deal with the same hefty gender baggage as their straight counterparts. Masculine men, regardless of their sexuality, have the necessary cultural capital to experiment more publicly and performatively with their gender. The rise of ostensibly straight actors and musicians — Jacob Elordi, Pedro Pascal, Harry Styles and the like — rocking a genderfuck garment on the red carpet or playing out queer (or aesthetically queer) relationships onstage and screen is evidence of this. For someone whose primary issue with the dogma of binary gender is its rigidity, I am excited at this new paragon of softer, experimental, whimsical masculinity: the babygirl.

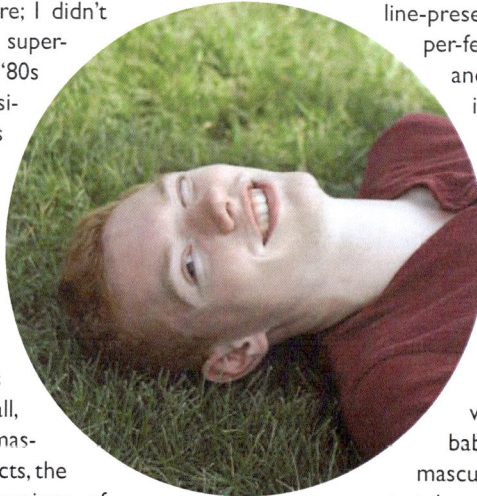

The "babygirl" is a rare, feminine term of endearment applied to men — often actors — who are largely traditionally masculine, yet strike a more whimsical pose in a photo, for example. In stark contrast to "sissy," "priss," or any number of other feminine terms derogatorily applied to men, "babygirl" is always a compliment. While the term's good-natured humor comes from the incongruity between the masculine-presenting subject and the hyper-feminine combo of "baby" and "girl," its connotation is always positive. Calling Pedro Pascal "babygirl" means he is endearing, warm, and isn't afraid to do what he wants. In other words, he isn't constrained by the straightjacket of traditional heteromasculinity. In much the same way as the contemporary babygirl, I have found my soft masculinity in the cracks and stretch-marks that form between my true self and the societally imposed mold of what a man is supposed to be. Those incongruities create interest and individuality. Stereotypically speaking, masculine traits are fundamental to my identity. I am ambitious, pragmatic, take-charge, and ultimately uncompromising in my pursuit of the things I want. But I will never sit through an entire sports game; I will never understand how a car works; I will never punch a wall, or master the art of the handshake-into-a-one-armed-hug, or even get really into fitness. These facts aren't compromising my sense of masculinity, but integral to redefining it. A babygirl need not know how to change a tire; they must simply be silly and cute while figuring it out.

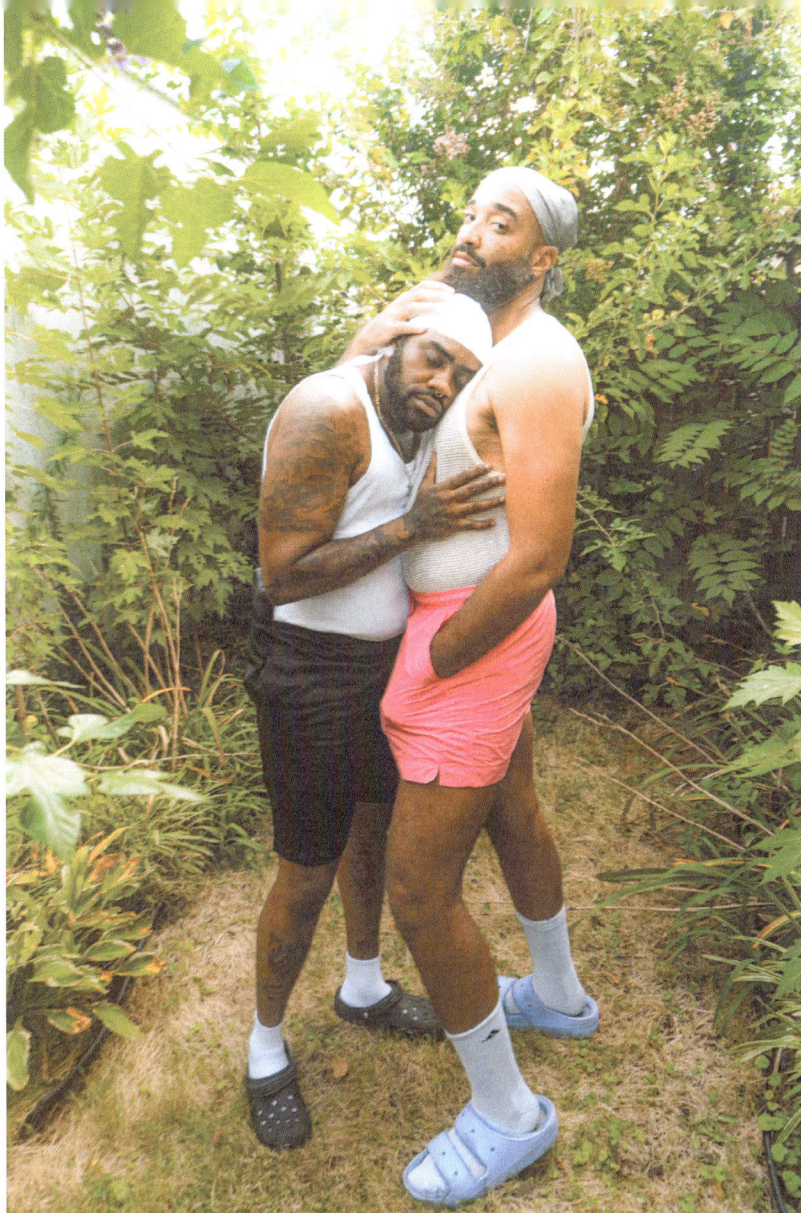

WHERE I WANNA BE

A VISUAL
STORTYELLING
OF BLACK LOVE,
INFIDELITY &
FORGIVENESS

Bearykah Shaw
they/them   @bearykahbadu

By using myself as the subject for most of my work, I began to uncover beauty in my own body as well as an appreciation for my blackness. My art deeply resonates with my emotions, and I try to encapsulate my feelings in my imagery.

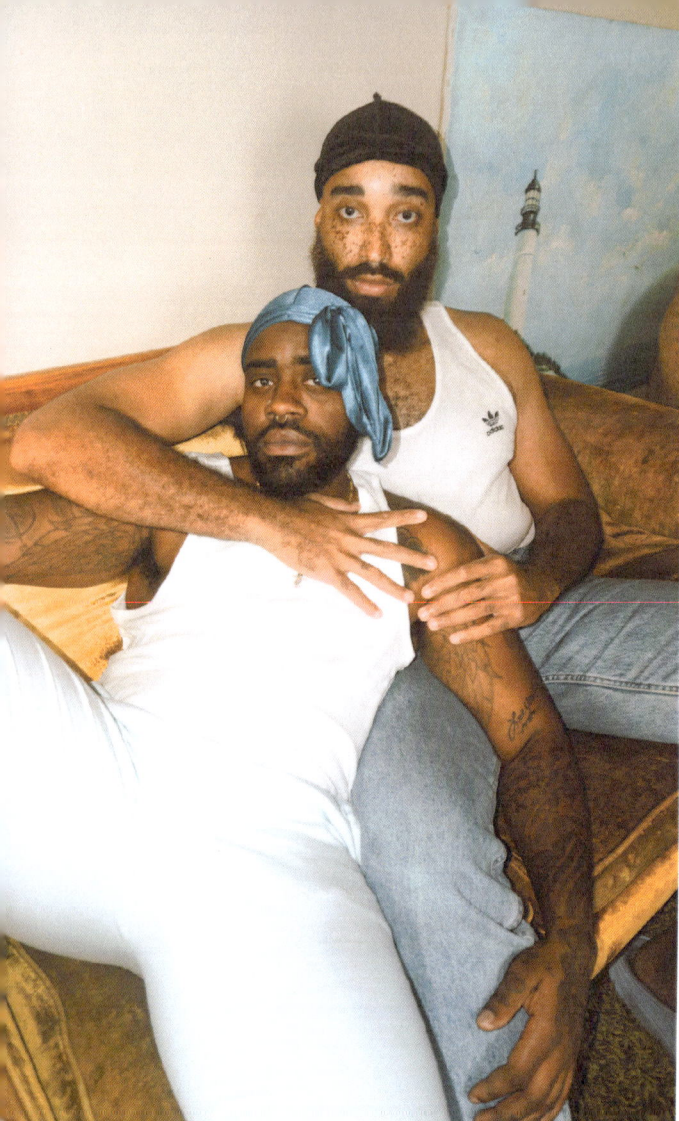

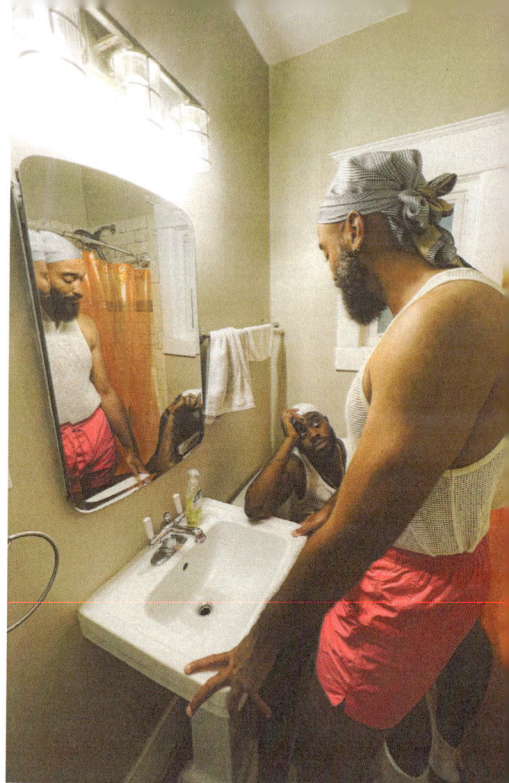

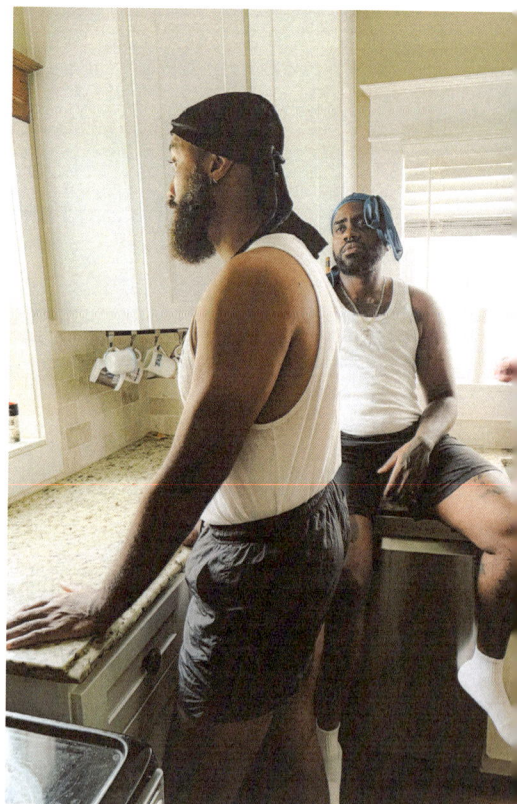

In this series, I explore the complex and fragile dynamics of relationships, particularly those between my best friend and I, who navigated the tumultuous waters of love, only to find ourselves entangled in a regrettable affair.

Through my work, I aim to convey the intricate emotions, the bittersweet memories, and the tragic aftermath of a connection that went astray, capturing the essence of human vulnerability and the blurred lines between friendship and romance.

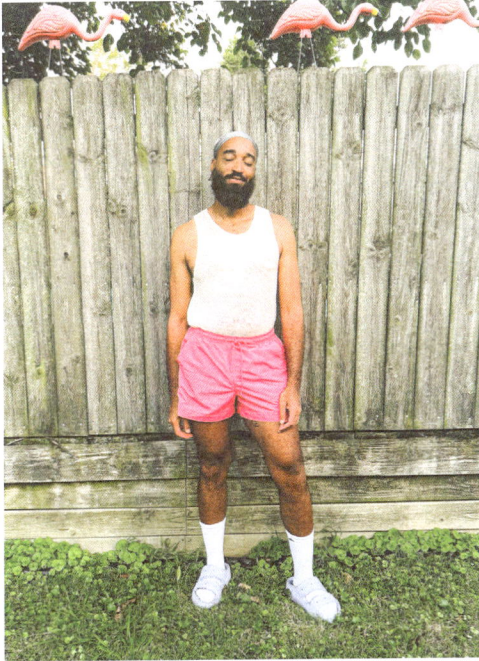
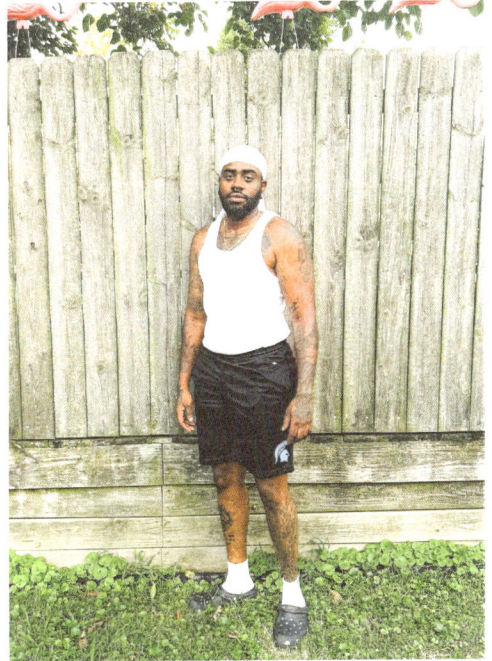
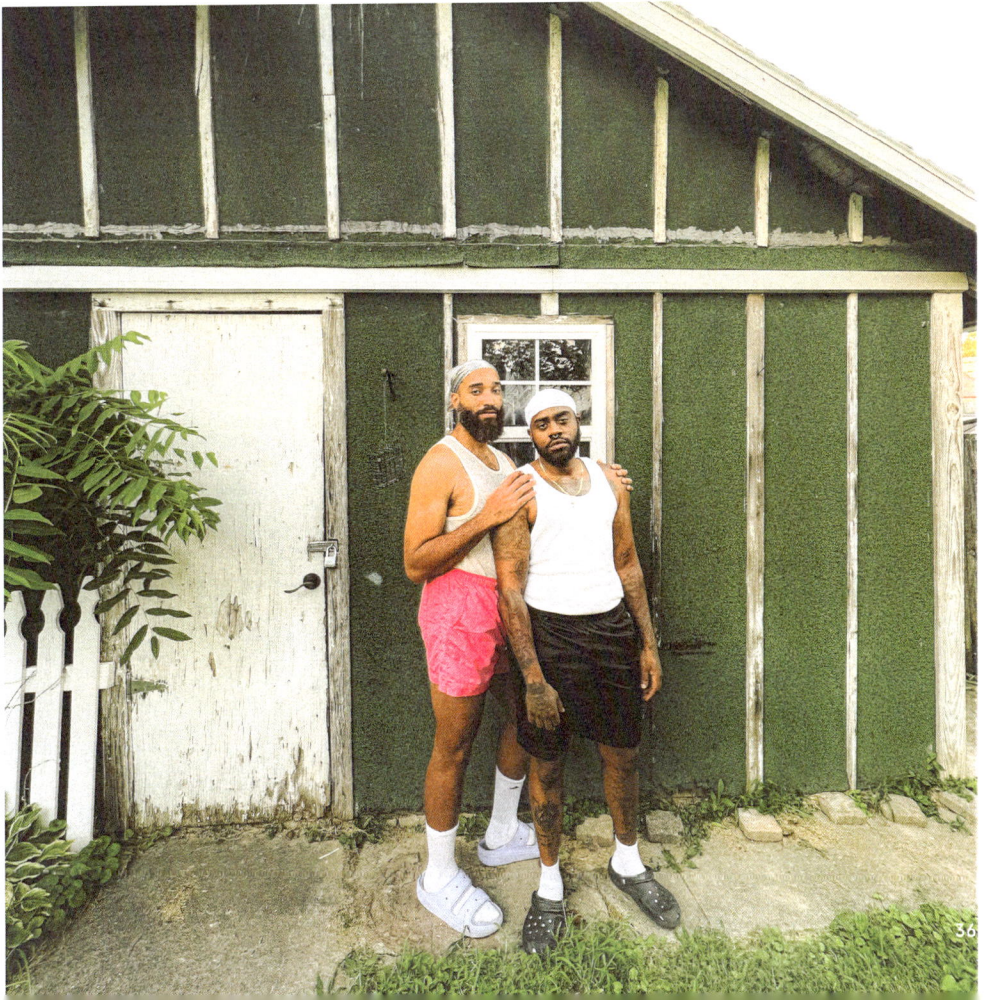

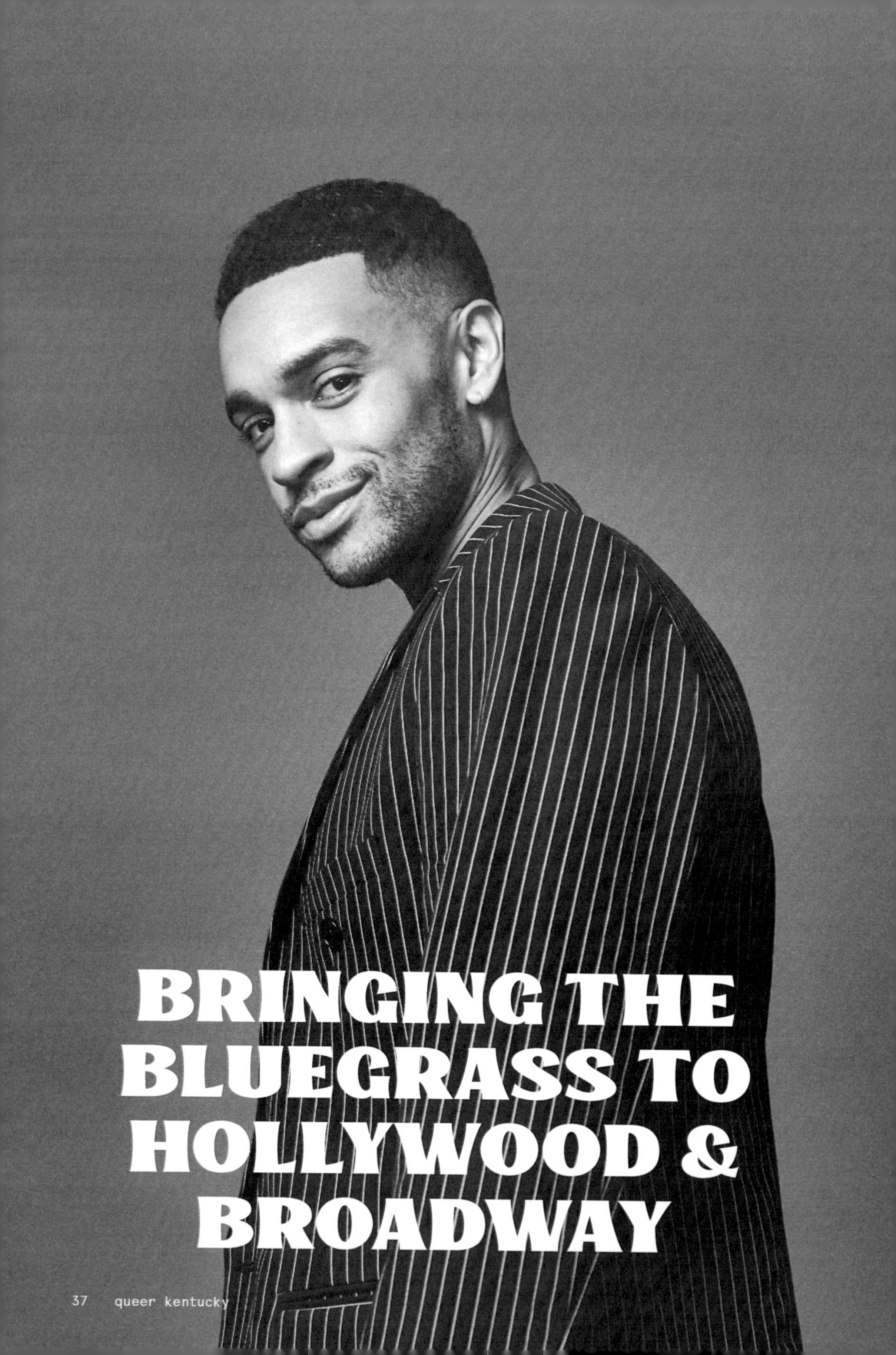

BRINGING THE BLUEGRASS TO HOLLYWOOD & BROADWAY

NOAH J. RICKETTS

he/him   @noahjrkts

I met Noah Ricketts through MySpace when that was one of the only ways to meet other queer kids. We were both young gay boys navigating life in Kentucky the best we could. We weren't besties and we didn't know each other that well, but for me at least, just knowing that another gay kid existed in the same city as me was enough to make me feel the small sense of community I craved. Throughout the years we followed each other's digital lives with occasional DMs of, "Congratulations!" after a professional triumph and some double tap likes here and there. I don't think we ever thought we'd be sitting together in a hotel lobby in the East Village of New York City in our 30s to discuss his blossoming entertainment career.

Spencer Jenkins

he/him   @spencerjenkss

photos by Josh Drake   he/him   @joshdrake.pdf | provided by Showtime

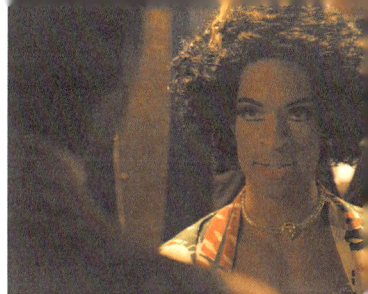

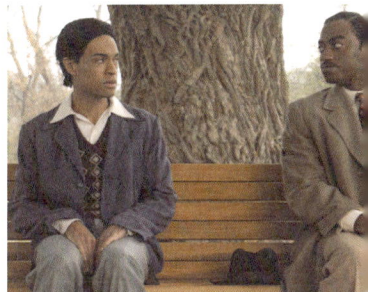

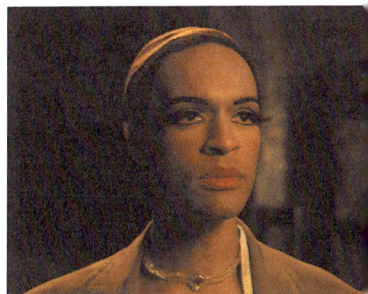

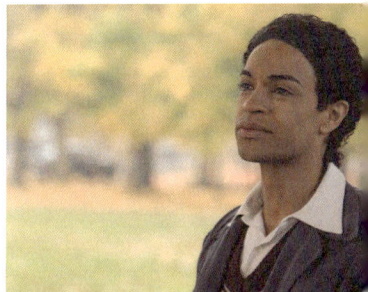

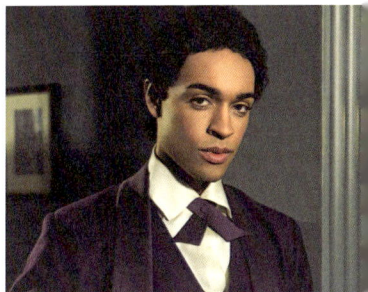

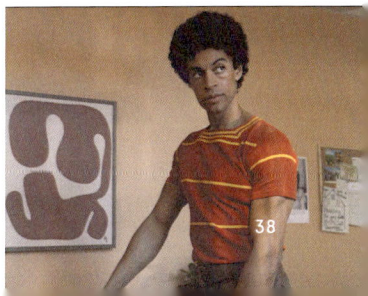

OF ALL THE KENTUCKIANS

who made it to the big and small screens, very few have been part of the LGBTQ+ community, much less challenge masculine ideals set forth by Hollywood and become a visible representation of Black queer men in the South — until now.

Noah Ricketts, Louisville, masterfully donned 1950s drag and 1980s swag as Frankie Hines in the Showtime political romance miniseries, *Fellow Travelers*. The show follows a group of men, led by Matt Bomer and Jonathan Bailey, through the Lavender Scare, the Vietnam War, and the AIDS Crisis.

In the show, Ricketts plays a drag queen performing in an underground queer nightclub in Washington D.C. as he navigates his place within the intersections of Blackness and queerness, all while falling in love with a man, played by Jelani Alladin, who's also struggling to find his own place in the world. Finding Frankie, he explains, proved to be a cathartic experience.

"I remember them shuffling me into a dress and leading me down this hallway and all of a sudden, the sea just parted," Ricketts recalls of his first day on set. "Everyone stares and looks at me. And I'm like, 'Oh God, what happened? What did I do?' And then I realize, 'Oh, they're staring at me because of how fabulous I look.'"

It was a defining moment for Ricketts. "You can hear a pin drop in that whole place," he continues. "In that moment, I realized the power of drag."

Queer shows like *Fellow Travelers* didn't exist when Ricketts was growing up in the Fern Creek area of Louisville, where he attended DuPont Manual High School (Youth Performing Art School). Now, he hopes it will "help queer content get off the ground" not only in Hollywood, but across the nation.

As a YPAS student, Ricketts bebopped around one of the more artistic and queer neighborhoods in Louisville — the Highlands. Now residing in the West Village neighborhood of New York City, he recalls the "rowdy girls" he got into trouble with in his teen years.

"We would go to my friend's house and sing on her mom's karaoke machine," he says with a laugh. "I've had many a night in Walmart parking lots, bonfires and in Waffle House."

In a 2000s era Kentucky, queer teens didn't have many outlets for connection with others like them. Ricketts says he didn't have a lot of queer friends growing up, but like many young gaybys, he was flush with wild straight girls.

"Those are my girls, my ride or dies that I would depend on and hang out with and who would console me. I really appreciated them," he says. "They were open and accepting of who I was at that time, even though I was figuring it out."

One of the shared experiences amongst young gay boys in the Bluegrass is being forced into sports that they don't want to play. Ricketts wound up playing soccer, though serendipity allowed his sports career to be cut short.

"I broke my arm a couple of weeks before I was supposed to go to soccer camp," he explains. "They don't allow injured children into sports at the YMCA, so I got shuffled off to the only place in Louisville that would take me, which was this musical theater summer camp called Broadway Bootcamp."

The snafu ended up being the catalyst to his life and career as an entertainer.

Broadway Bootcamp was a game-changer. It was the first time he was surrounded by people who were acting, singing, and dancing — a world he'd never before experienced before. He became obsessed with theater and would stay up late watching any Tony Award performances on YouTube he could find.

"I was reading plays, going to dance lessons, voice lessons — anything I could do to get my hands on art," he says of those days. But there was a limit to his dreams.

Ricketts knew that Kentucky wasn't necessarily the place he needed to grow as a queer performer, so he took a risk and dropped out of YPAS to uproot his life for Interlochen Center for the Arts in Michigan. After he graduated from the arts boarding school, he jumped right back to the Ohio River Valley at the University of Cincinnati's prestigious musical theater program. Four intense years there led him directly to auditions on Broadway in New York City.

"It was pretty crazy because as a person studying musical theater for so long, to finally be

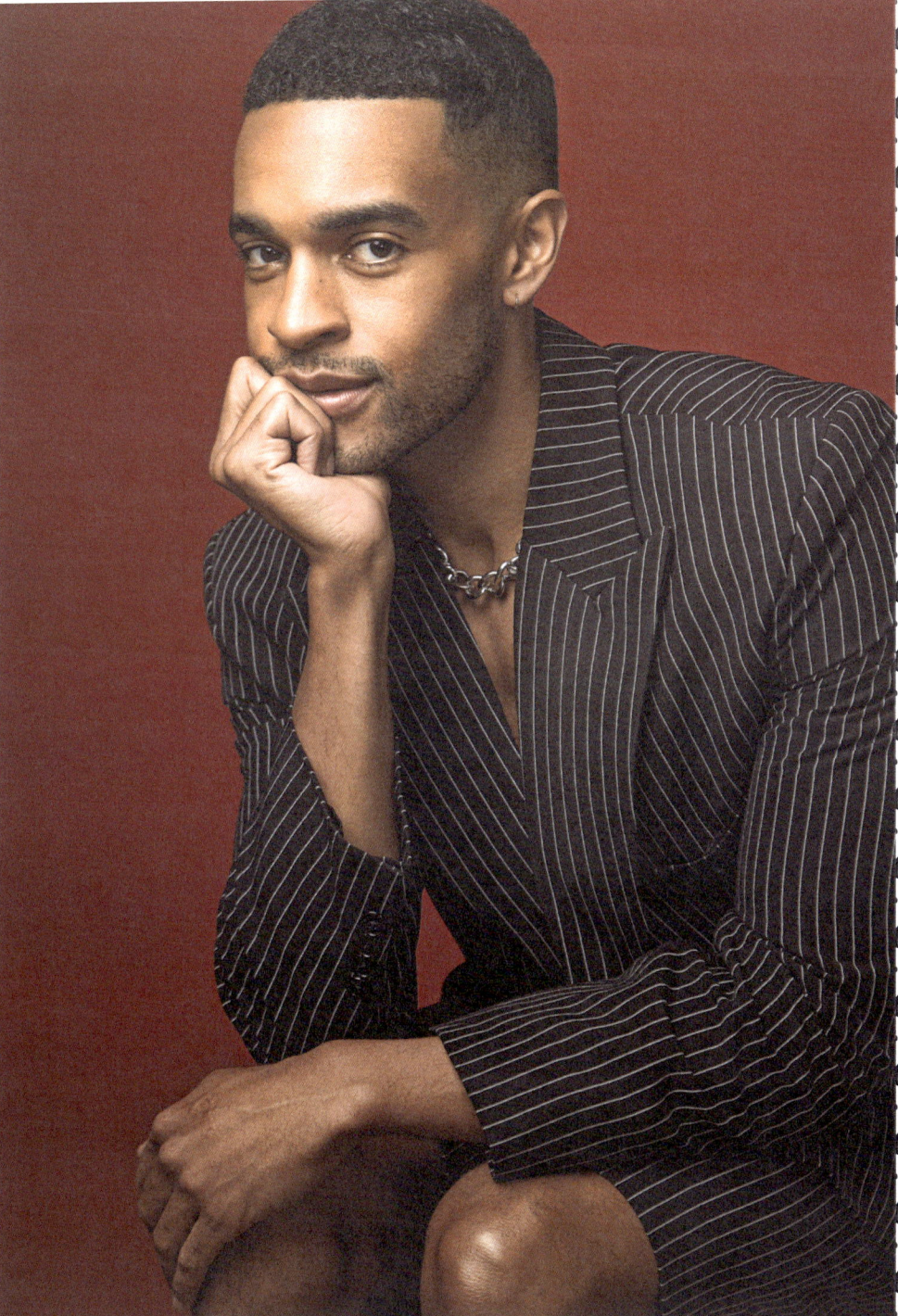

In that moment, I realized the power of dra
In that moment, I realized the power of dra
In that moment, I realized the power of dra
In th   dra
In th   dra
In th   dra
In th   dra
In th   dra
In th   dra
In th   dra
In th   dra
In th   dra
In th   dra
In th   dra
In th   dra
In th   dra
In th   dra
In th   dra
In th   dra
In th   dra
In th   dra
In th   dra
In that moment, I realized the power of dra
In that moment, I realized the power of dra
In that moment, I realized the power of dra

thrown into the world and be auditioning for proper shows was such a surreal experience," Ricketts says.

The hard work paid off. Soon after landing in the Big Apple, Ricketts starred on Broadway as Drifter in *Beautiful, The Carole King Musical* and Kristoff in *Frozen* as well as shows like Dreamgirls, *Hello, Dolly!, Tarzan and La Cage aux Folles*. This Spring, he's set to star in *The Great Gatsby* as Nick Carraway, alongside Jeremy Jordan and Eva Noblezada.

Frozen is also where Ricketts met his *Fellow Travelers'* costar, Jelani Alladin, who plays Frankie Hines' love interest, Marcus Hooks. The two were "partners in crime" on set and barely got through a take without laughing.

"Noah is the truest personification of a gem. He is the result of hard work and explosive talent, existing simultaneously in a vessel filled with compassion, empathy, and game," Aladdin, said. "I can't wait to witness what great works he will continue to give this world."

It was his starring role in *Frozen* that gave Ricketts pause, knowing that he broke new ground playing a Black Disney Prince. Even now, it makes him emotional.

"I didn't realize how important that moment was until I reflect on it now," he says. "I remember having all these young Black boys waiting for me after the show and at first I was like, 'Oh, this is a mistake' or 'They must be waiting for someone else.' And then I realized, 'Oh, no, they came

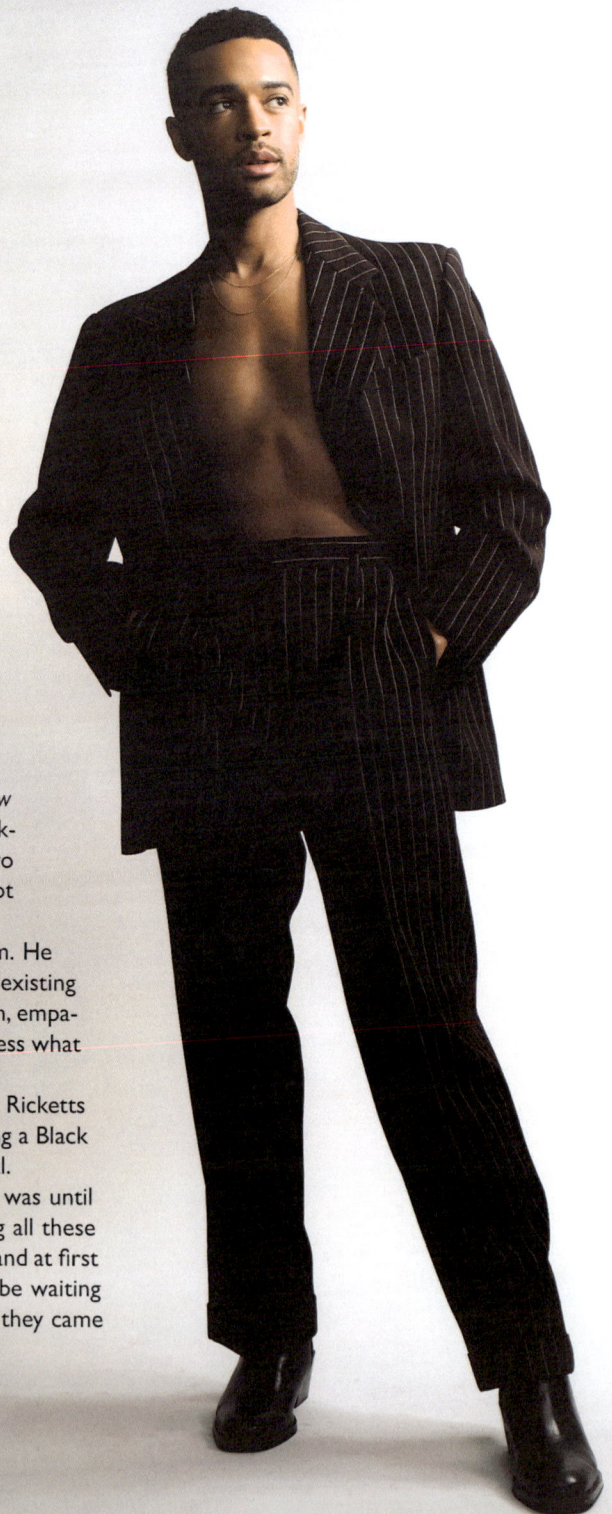

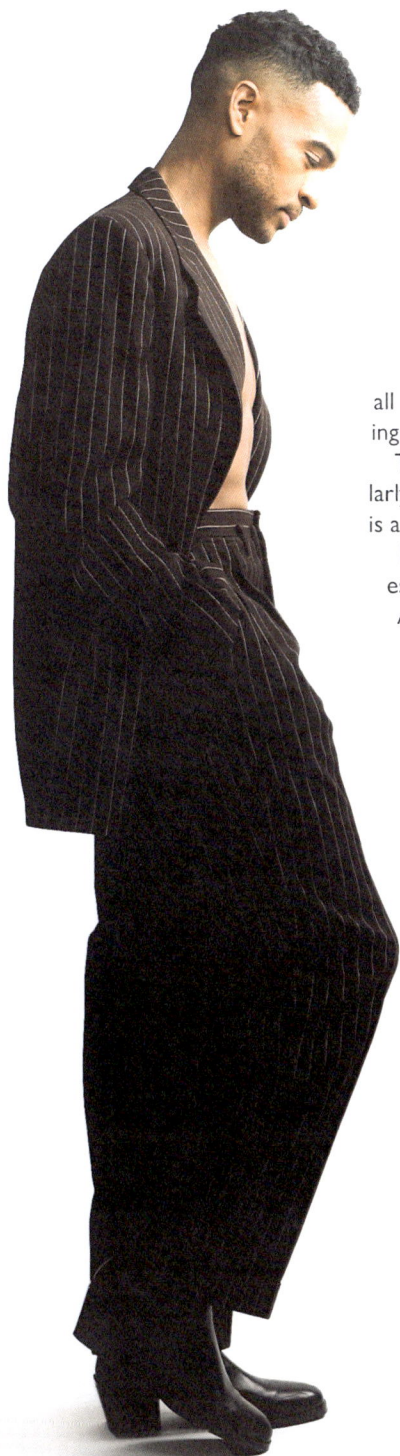

all this way to see me.' I realized for the first time in my life, I was making change and using my art for good."

The moment made him realize "how powerful" art can be, particularly to queer Black kids. "At that moment, I decided, this is what this is all about."

Ricketts holds the same adoration for *Fellow Travelers*, which in essence is a visual history of the traumatic realities of the AIDS crisis. As he points out, queer people are taking notice of the message the show is putting out.

"I've gotten a lot of messages from people in the older gay community, just saying thank you, because I feel like they've just been seen for the first time in decades and now I'm getting messages from the younger community," he says. "They're DMing me on Instagram or responding to TikToks. I love it."

As Ricketts heads back to Broadway, the rest of the world can expect more groundbreaking projects from him — as well as some grassroots community work — in the coming years.

Recently, he's been working with Louisville native filmmaker, Imani N. Dennison, on a project detailing the life of a famous Black jockey, Isaac Burns Murphy. Ricketts and Dennison want to make the film in Louisville and involve the community during its production. He is also working to reestablish the very same Broadway Bootcamp that took him in as a young teen and ignited his love for art and music. It's certainly a full circle moment.

"My accessibility to the arts as a young person is why I am here today," he says. "I'd like to continue that pipeline from Louisville to Broadway [by bringing] in New York's best talents to the Bluegrass state. It's a win-win for everyone."

WHEN WILL I MEET MYSELF?

Simone Jackson

she/he/they   @odditiques

This piece depicts a person having a gender identity crisis on their kitchen floor, and they're trying to do their makeup to feel better, however, their reflection is skewed so they cannot properly see themselves. This is to symbolize that they are confused about who they are. This is demonstrated to onlookers of the piece, as they are allowed to look into this intimate moment, and see off to the side what the figure is seeing of themselves. However, the person is too focused on their present self, they do not see the Ox behind them in the fridge, symbolizing patience and strength. They also do not see the mulberries in the foreground that represent abundance and growth. These are all signs of their future, that if they are to just accept themselves as they are, they can grow to be a stronger person.

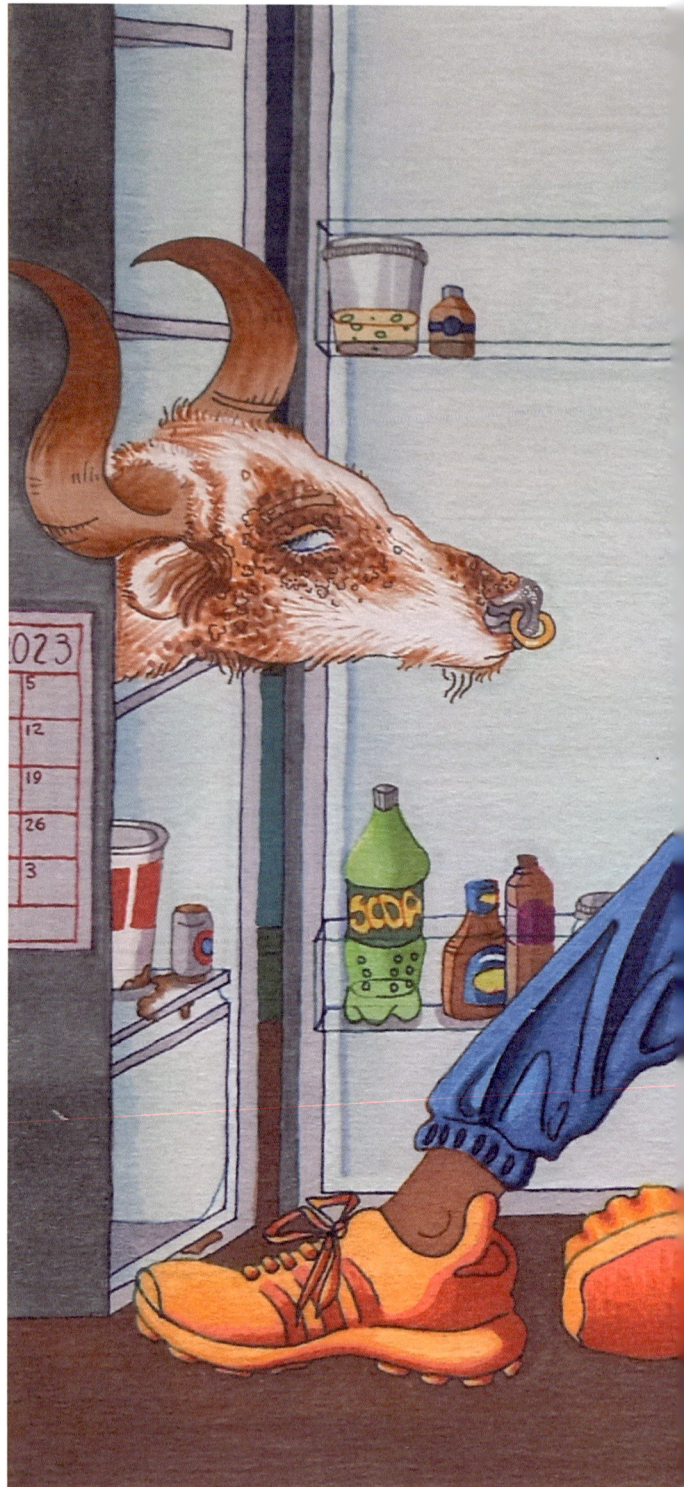

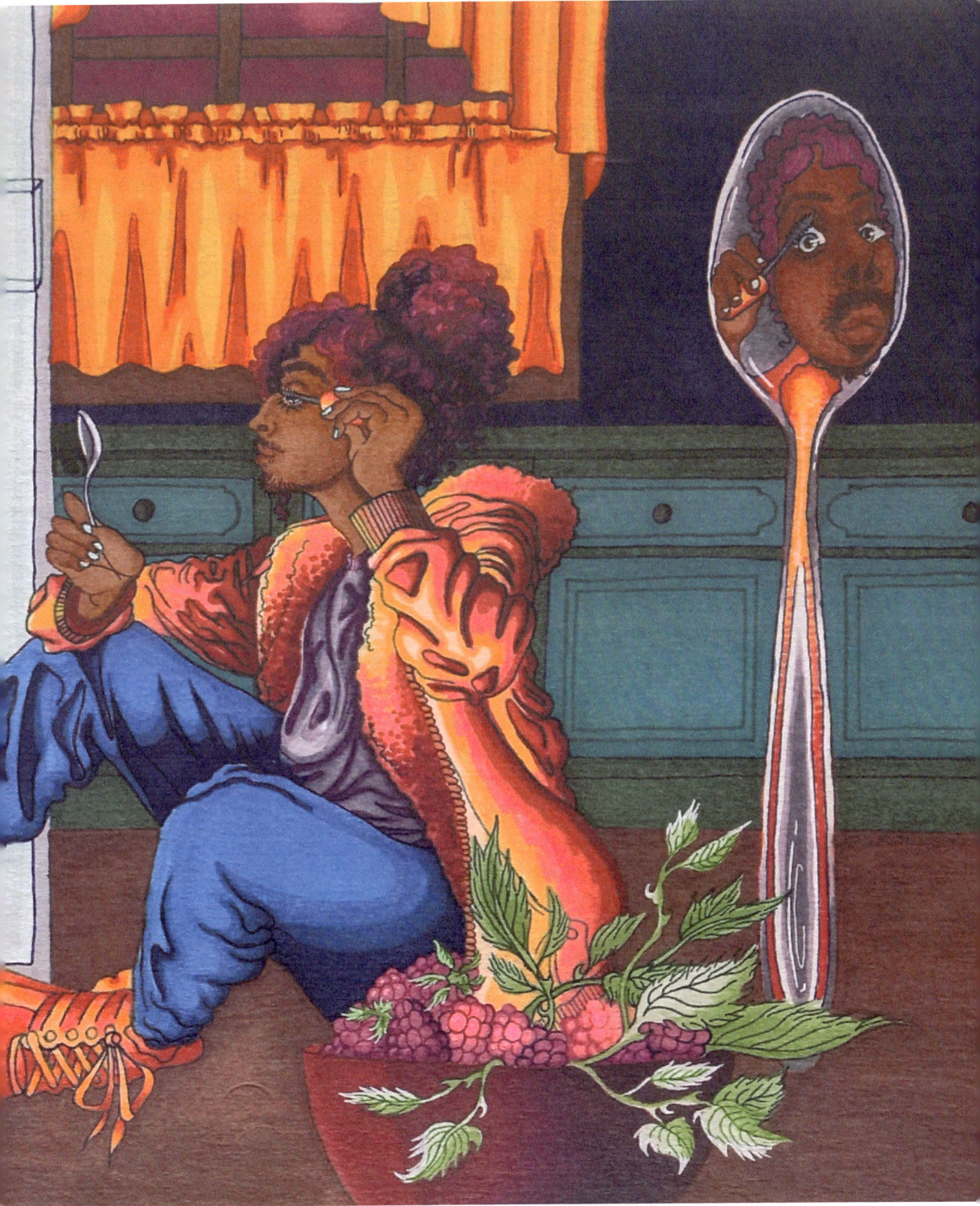

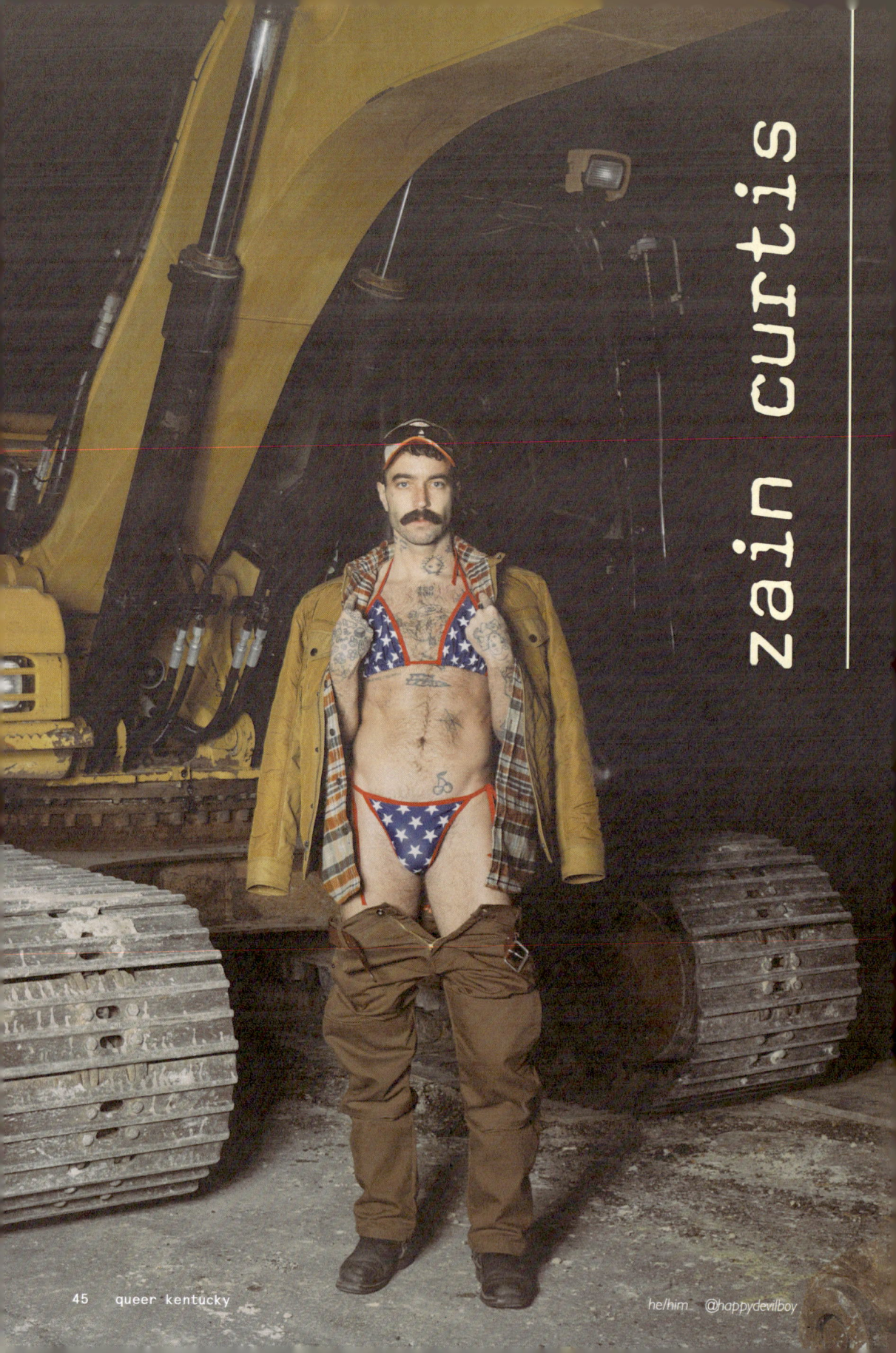

zain curtis

I Will Follow You to BG 'Cause That's What Us Boys Are For

BOWLING GREEN BORN ARTIST CREATES UNCENSORED PLATFORM FOR QUEER CREATIVES

Spencer Jenkins
he/him @spencerjenkss

In 2022, I stumbled upon an Instagram post of a sun-kissed bronze, tatted, and otteresque artist, Zain Curtis. He had recently gained notoriety from screen printing T-shirts with blood infused paint to raise awareness of the homophobic blood ban in the United States. With my "pick-me" energy, I feverishly DMed "I have to write about you for Queer Kentucky." Unbeknown to me, Curtis is a Bluegrass-bred boy and was happy to join me in getting back to his Bowling Green roots.

If you're a queer person who fancies erotic art, raunchy porn, drag culture, and controversy, then you've gotten your gooey thumb stuck onto a kink-inspired photo of creator Zain Curtis.

Curtis, also known by his Instagram handle @Happydevilboy or his magazine, SENSITIVE CONTENT @sensitivecontentmag, has built an extensive career in queer media — and he loves creating media around all things sex, specifically kink and fetish.

"I always found it so mind-blowing that we have the most fucked up relationship with what is the most natural to us — blood, urine, cum, menstruation, sex, shitting, vomit — like if everything else in the world disappeared and it was just our bodies, these would be all we know," said the SENSITIVE CONTENT magazine founder.

When Curtis began creating art on these topics in a social media-focused world, he was met with post removals, shadow bans, and full account bans. He also started noticing a trend: queer creatives were constantly getting scrubbed and censored from the Internet.

"Most things I created were things purely to be viewed on social media," the sex industry entrepreneur said. "I didn't keep copies of it, so all of my photos of that time in my life, the things I made, and everything about it were just gone forever," he said. "People are like, 'Oh, what you post on the internet lasts forever,' but that's so not true."

He adds that Meta, the parent brand of Instagram has bulldozed any competing apps that would be a suitable outlet for his art and that banks and payment processors have the overall decision on what rules apps have to follow if they want to be used with mass audiences.

SENSITIVE CONTENT was born out of a reaction to the censoring of queer artists. Curtis describes the magazine as a "visual showcase of artwork and photos by LGBTQIA+ creators that have been removed or restricted by social media platforms."

"[SENSITIVE CONTENT] came together naturally, and before I knew it, I found so many cool artists going through the same issues with social media," he said. "It's a baby to me. I'm still figuring out what the future of it can be, but right now, it's been a fun side project when I'm not working on my own things."

At first, the Happy Devil Boy painter said the magazine was purely about removed posts, but he realized a rift existed between queer readers' ideas of what they would see and Curtis' ideas of what SENSITIVE CONTENT was about.

Curtis wants the magazine to be an unbiased and offline space for any and all ideas by queer and trans people, not a bubble of similar thinking.

"It's hard to figure that out and make that a sellable thing to different types of people because no one really wants to listen to anyone that they don't fully agree with anymore" he said. "There's a formula to it that I haven't harnessed yet, but I'm excited for its growth."

In his magazine, Curtis and his writers cover topics of all sorts: gooning, trans bodies, public sex, political activism and more. With the tagline, "Make the Algorithm Cum," the featured uncensored creators certainly don't edge their audience for long.

Curtis believes that people love collecting things like tangible magazines — something the internet hasn't taken away from us.

"It is a different feeling to hold content you enjoy in your hands versus seeing it on a screen," he said. "There's much more attachment to it, and I think it lingers in people's minds more."

Although Curtis may be known well for his provocative nudey magazine during this portion of his 15 minutes of fame, the well-rounded artist has been in the game since an early age.

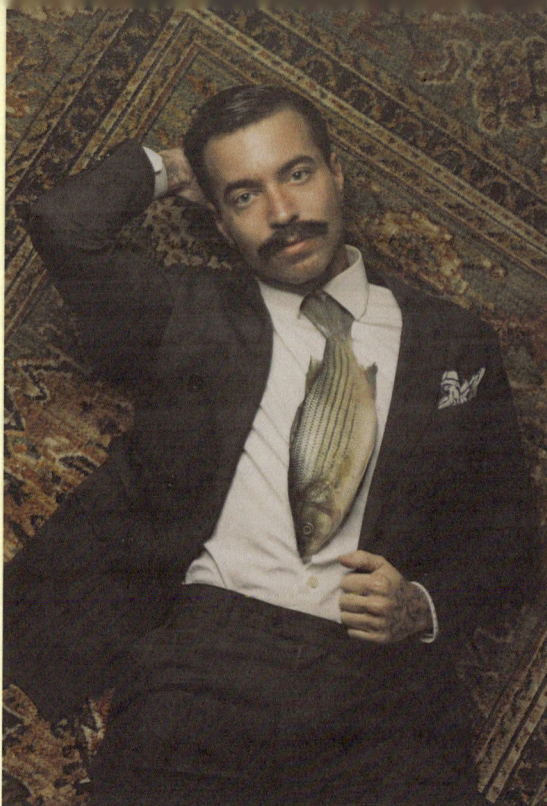

After leaving his hometown of Bowling Green, Kentucky., he landed where many midwestern and southern gays land: Chicago. The Windy City is where Curtis went to film school, began DJing and curating events, and started his first publication, Teen Witch Magazine.

"[It] was what I called an underground teen magazine that featured all trans and queer artists and social media personalities of the time. It was basically promoting my friends, but I made it look like a teeny-bopper magazine and made fold-out posters, sticker sheets, and puzzles for them," he said. "It was like a way of finding cool people and instantly idolizing them. I think SENSITIVE CONTENT is like the adult version of that."

One of Curtis' projects went viral in 2022 when he used gay men's blood to protest the blood ban on queer men. In a statement on his Instagram Curtis said, "No, really. Printed with ink infused with the blood of gay men. Using screen printing ink from Stuart Semple × Mother's GAY BLOOD collection."

Bold and controversial pieces are at the core of Curtis' entrepreneurial journey — so is his personality. He said his favorite aspect of being a founder is the independence. And who could blame him?

"If I want to fuck off I can and most likely will, probably to a fault," he said. "I can create my own world and make something from nothing. That's got to be a skill within itself."

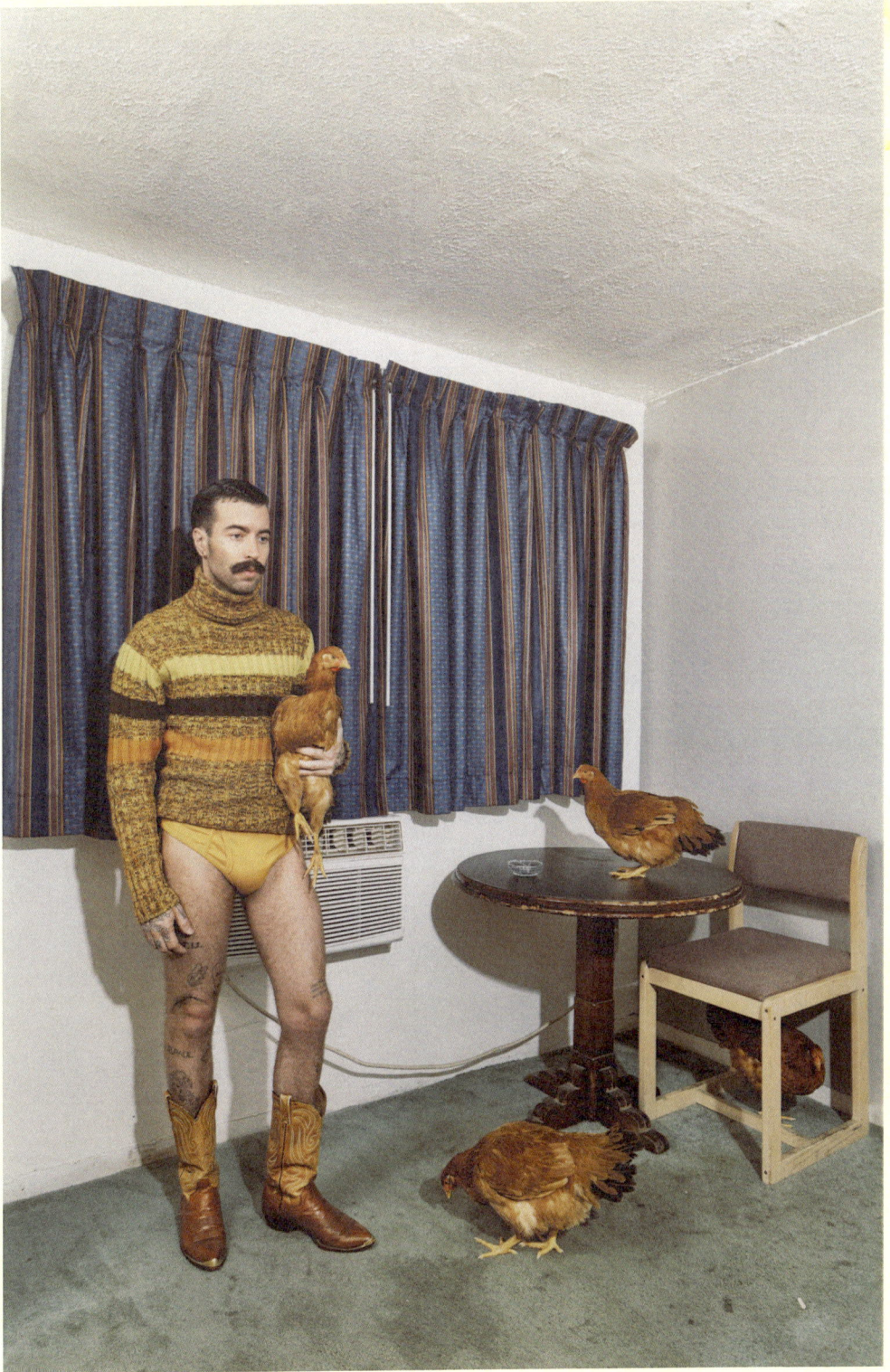

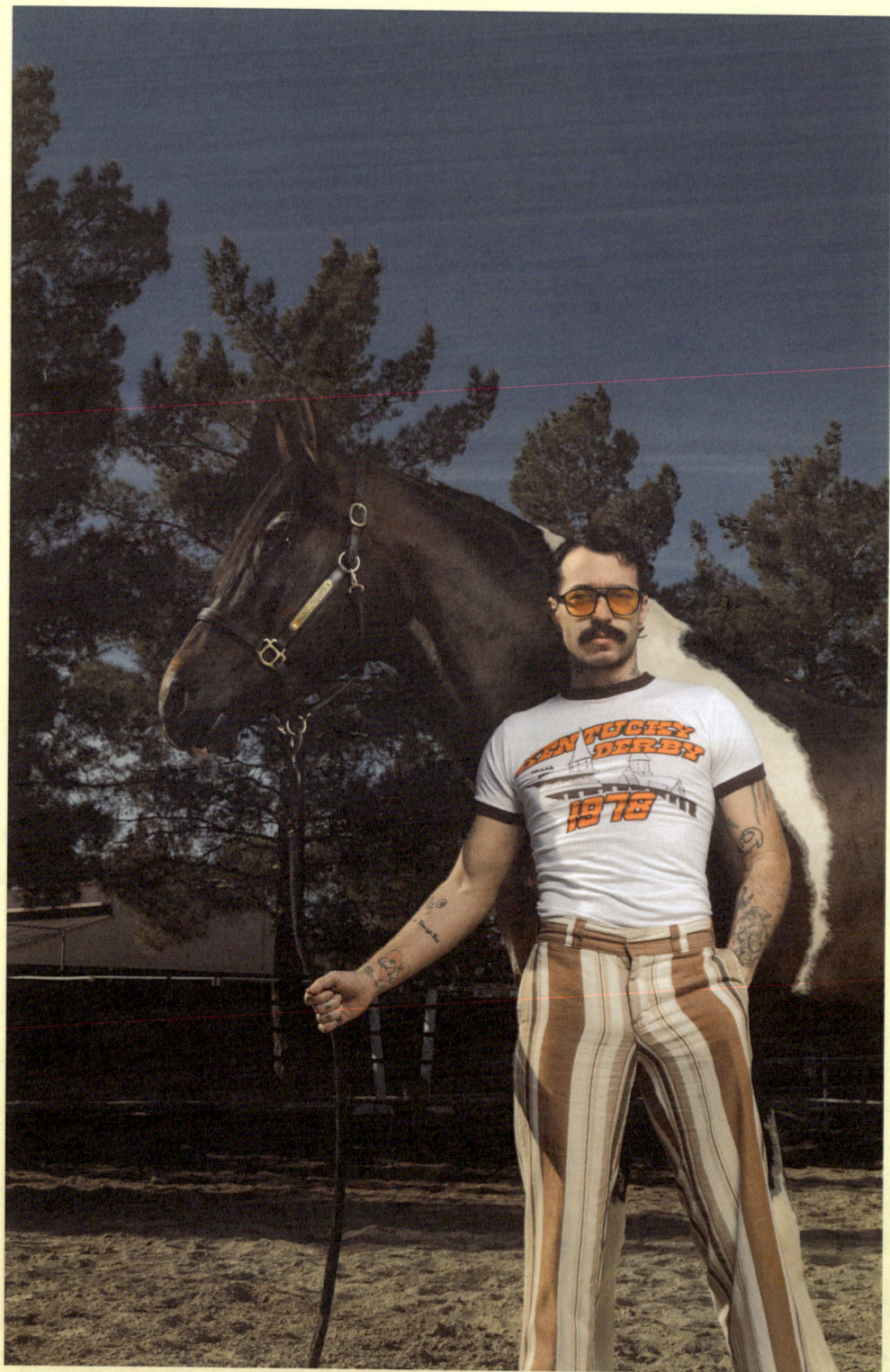

So yes, I miss home. I miss everything.

Does Kentucky play a role in any of your creations?

I'm really getting into country music, the Southern lifestyle, and cowboy culture and feeling more involved with something I basically ran away from. I spent enough time away that I can appreciate what it is now. I look back at growing up there, and I'm very inspired to write a book about it. I'm hoping to start that this year between everything else. I thought about staying in Kentucky for the summer to really feel it. It would be so emotional, but I see it all. I have to get the story out of me. I also have to do my banjo lessons, so we will see what I have the time for.

Sometimes, it's not what was around me that I get inspired by, but the feeling of when I lived there. It might have been mostly not having to pay for shelter, but there was such a sense of non-urgency that I really tried to hang onto. Like "I will get there when I get there" kind of feeling. The dicking around town with no purpose, but the purpose was just to have fun. Like the most mundane things were my favorite memories, I don't know if I'm trying to recreate that or push my thoughts away for a moment to live. I'm always fucking worried about something now though, it's hard.

Do you miss home?

I miss everything. I'm a very nostalgic person. I miss my exes, my old friendships, even the shitty living situations. I constantly live in the past; it's the only thing that calms me, it seems. I miss Kentucky and my family a lot, but every time I go back, it's like a shell of what I felt there before. Most people I knew moved away or grew up and had their own families. It's a weird feeling. I chase those old feelings all the time.

When I visited my mom last, I went around town and just visited all the old places I would hang out at. I went and saw a movie alone at the theater I used to work at and just had crazy memories flood my mind. Jackass was my favorite TV show, so my friends would do the absolute worst pranks on each other. One was "borrowing" deer piss from the Wal-Mart hunting section and chasing each other and splashing it on our clothes. One time, I opened my car door and was knocked off my feet by the smell. My friend poured so many bottles of it all over my seats. I never got that smell out of my car. I went to work, and they sent me home because of the smell on me. I drove to the parking lot and was like, "Aww, that's where my car was parked when that happened." So yes, I miss home. I miss everything.

How has the west coast treated you?

I really love the West; it's somewhere I never imagined I would be, but it's indescribable what the desert has done for me and my mental health. I was so painstakingly depressed when I moved to LA; everything seemed like such a challenge and not a ladder I even wanted to climb. I'm so happy I made the choice to live in the desert and basically got to start over. It was the first time I started to feel that Kentucky feeling of non-urgency again. I needed to be alone and recalibrate what I was doing and wanted to do.

I recently moved to Las Vegas. Just because it's cheaper than California and there's a bit more opportunity than living in the middle of nowhere. It doesn't feel like home, but a rest stop along the way. It is inspiring, the people are really fucking weird and such characters. It's so trashy; I fit right in. I have in my head that I'll live on a little ranch in a trailer outside the city, just far enough to see the glow of the strip. Have chickens, a horse and two goats. That's all I want is two goats.

SCULPTED FLESH

Xander Jarvis   *He/They*   *@xander.does.art*

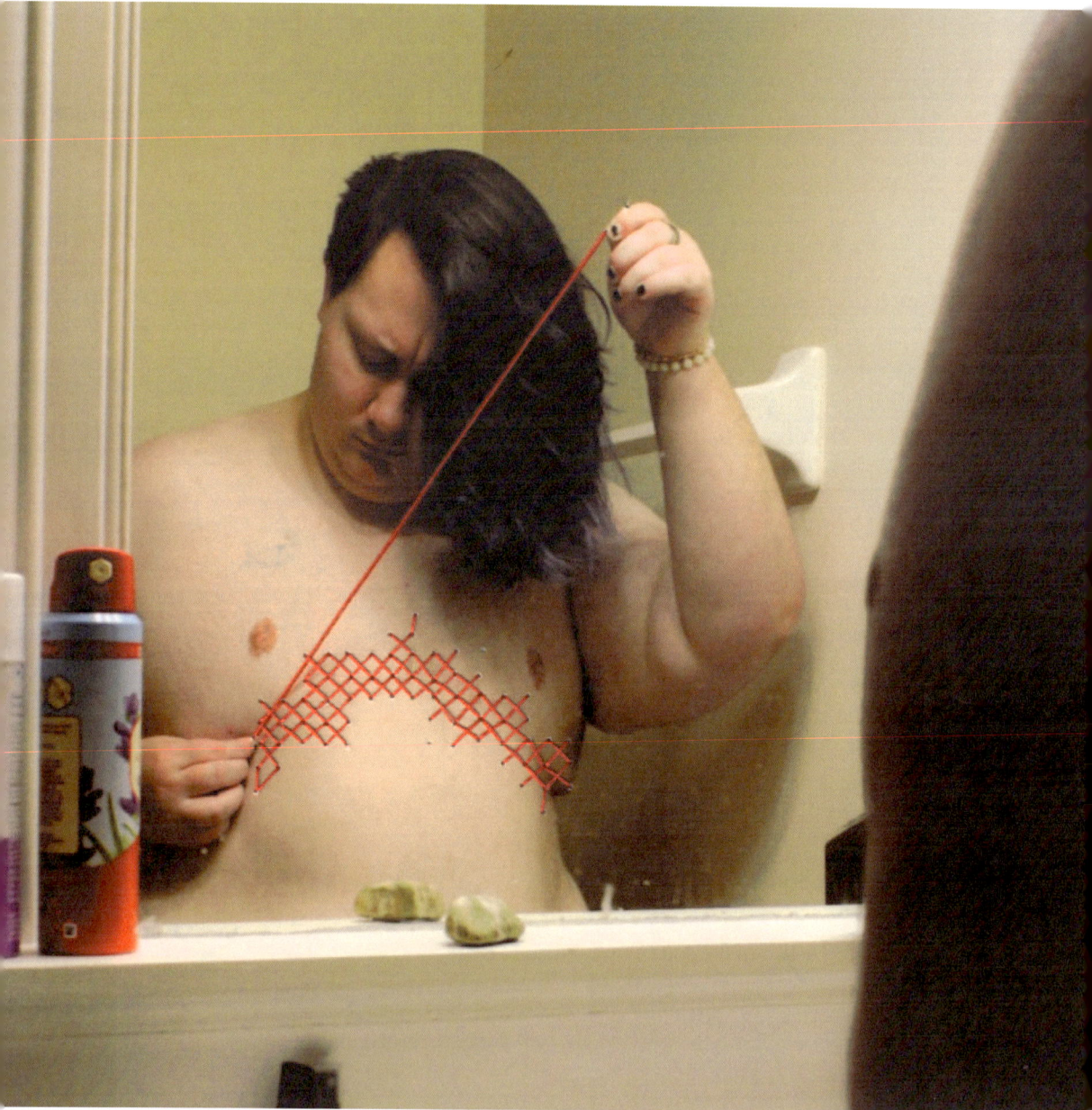

photos by Xander Jarvis   He/they

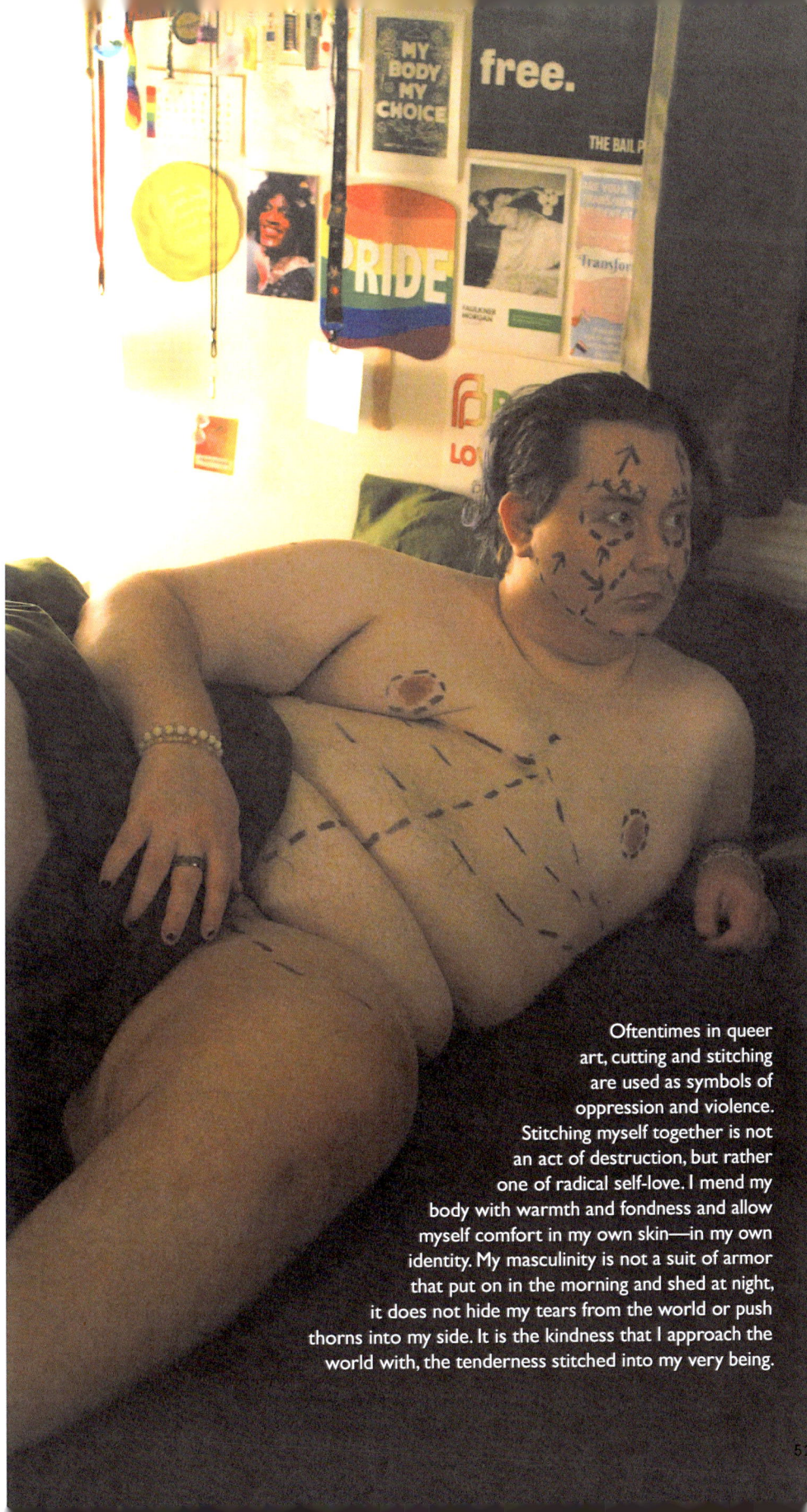

Oftentimes in queer art, cutting and stitching are used as symbols of oppression and violence. Stitching myself together is not an act of destruction, but rather one of radical self-love. I mend my body with warmth and fondness and allow myself comfort in my own skin—in my own identity. My masculinity is not a suit of armor that put on in the morning and shed at night, it does not hide my tears from the world or push thorns into my side. It is the kindness that I approach the world with, the tenderness stitched into my very being.

I spy a Sky Dancer, a Doodle Bear, a Barbie from '59,
Five pigs, a beauty sponge, and ...*Baby One More Time*;

A neon pink Prada mule, a distant post-Covid utopia,
A creature named Laa-Laa, and lingering internalized homophobia.

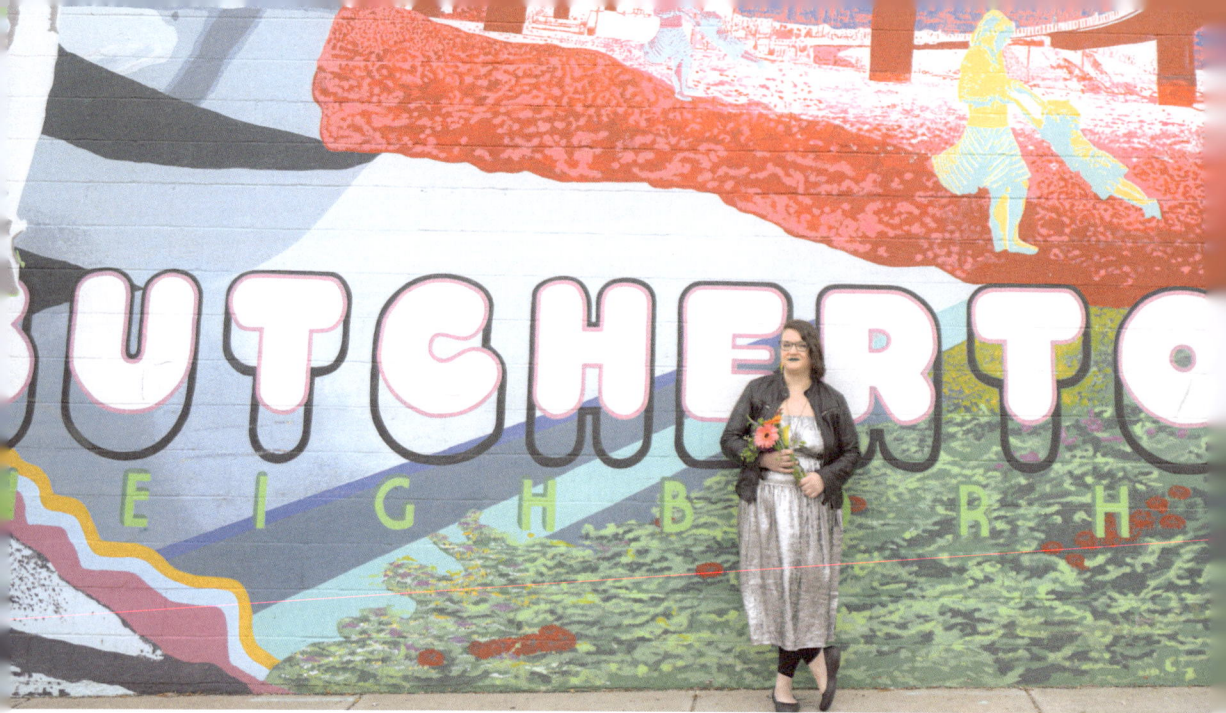

LEE INITIATIVE LUNCH BREAK

Ashlee Martinis   @ChefAshleeMartinis

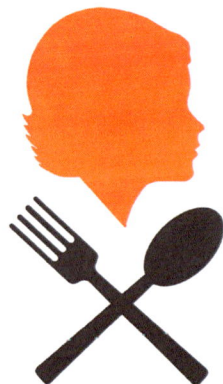

"WHY DO YOU HAVE TO ACT LIKE A GUY ALL THE TIME?"

My first boyfriend asked me this after I won at video games, board games - definitely after getting better paychecks. But he was also critical of everything "feminine" I did, like spending too much money on beauty products or clothes. There was a constant toxic balancing of my "threatening" masculinity and my "exasperating" femininity, and it made my head spin. Coupled with lifelong insinuations of being gay from outsiders, you have a recipe for self-denial. I was in an abusive cis relationship for 12 years.

I liked playing sports when I was younger, but had no interest in watching them on TV. I love being outdoors but hate getting dirty. I work on my own cars but want to be a Suzy Homemaker. These contradictions, emphasized by gendered stereotypes, built me up to believe that no one would want me because I wasn't enough of one or the other.

When I finally realized that I was gay all along —pansexual attracted to femmes—I began to build friendships and community with people who share the way I would ultimately begin to see the world: tomboy femmes, gay men, lesbians, and straight geeks.

I am now a chef. As many of you know, fine dining is a male-dominated industry. I've spent so much time in kitchens drowning in toxic masculinity, dirty jokes, and sexual harassment/discrimination. Despite this, I was still trying to be "one of the guys" - to be accepted and not seen as weak. Femininity is not an asset in

photos by Jon Cherry   he/him   @jonpcherry

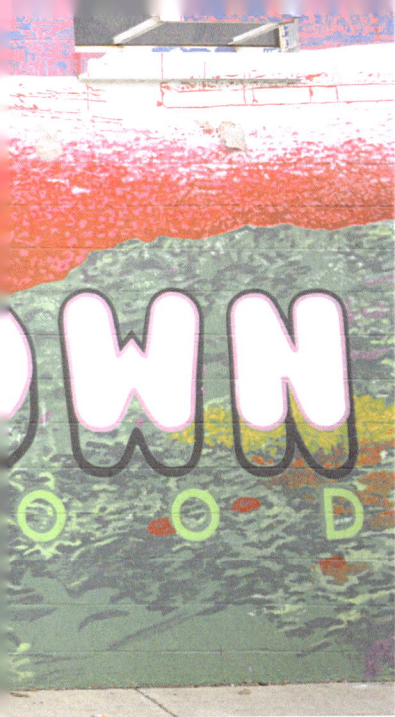

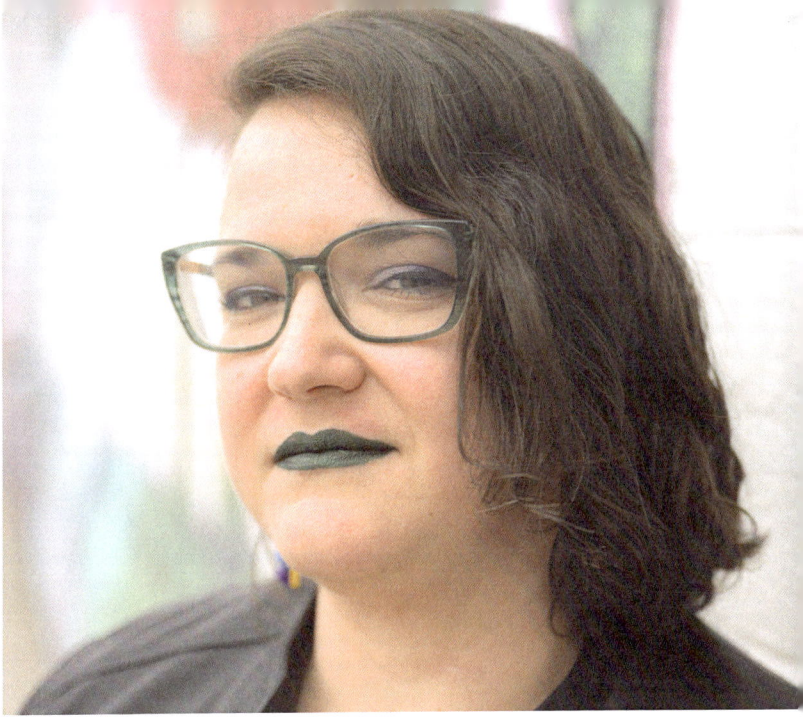

the kitchen, and many women chefs suppress it to succeed.

In January of 2020, a few months before the COVID-19 quarantine hit, my brother killed himself. My brother was also queer and had been struggling with his bisexuality - what that meant for his masculinity - for years. My grief and my anger were massive wounds. I had not been tapped to become the chef of my restaurant yet, but it was on the table. Before I had time to make a decision on how to express my grief, I was told,

> *"You can take time off, but I know you – you'll want to tough it out and work."*

Thinking that strong behavior was expected of me, I made the decision to work through my loss. Crying at work was seen as a liability, so I held it in. I transformed it to anger instead.

Then the world decided to end, and quarantine began. I worked my ass off, never really mourning or showing the emotions that I know now that I had every right to show. I followed the "Bro Code" of "Harden the Fuck Up" and was eventually tapped to be the new Chef. My new crown weighed heavy on my head.

Often, we save softer expressions for our family or our partners. But dating as a chef can be tough, due to lack of time and energy. Women chefs often end up dating within those same toxic professional circles. I was hurt many times by my own expectations. My dating choices were usually other line cooks with the same schedules who, instead of seeing our commonality, saw my successes as competition to their own careers. Ultimately, I wasn't girlfriend material, because they also saw me as one of the boys.

In 2022, I decided to leave my job in Virginia - moving 3000 miles cross-country to California. My grief from my brother's death became compounded when our mother passed away. I was not happy at my job, my health was suffering, and I had ghosted my last situationship. In California, I decided that I was giving up on dating.

Then I met her.

My girl is a trans woman who has spent most of her life being forced to be a "dude's dude." Our first date was San Francisco Pride. I spent most of it not really knowing yet that I was actually gay. She was also in the restaurant industry - my expo to be exact. She was a Jill of All Trades - lead server, bartender, bar back, and expo - and one of the hardest workers I'd ever seen. I found that incredibly attractive. She had recently put in her two weeks notice to go back to school, and I thanked my lucky stars that I had gotten up the courage to ask her out before I missed my chance.

The area of California where we lived was conservative, and being queer was still risky in areas. But I encouraged her to be herself, and we traveled throughout the Bay Area, attempting to be more open about our queerness. In turn, she allowed me to be as openly masculine or feminine as I wanted to be. But I still struggled with gender roles.

Did I need to be the "guy" or the "girl" in this relationship? The end answer surprised me, even though I think my brain knew all along. There is no male/female role. Only love, responsibility, loyalty, and a belief in each other—that we can survive and thrive in any situation. I've spent most of our relationship being the breadwinner, due to her school obligations, but I know now that that doesn't need to be associated with masculinity. Being ready to defend her if someone is cruel is not toxic masculinity; it's support and care.

I've ended up in Louisville, and I'm currently working for a wonderful female chef. Being back in my beloved South is wonderful and terrifying at the same time.

I don't feel like my new family can go back to my home state of Tennessee, due to their current laws prohibiting trans people from existing. I know legislative powers in Kentucky are trying to accomplish the same thing. But I still left California to secure us a future in a space where we can be freely queer and also have opportunities to succeed and chase our dreams. We are both working towards getting away from conservative areas that stifle her own femininity - areas that try to force her back into a masculine box.

"I am 40 years old. It turns out that I can hold space for masculinity and femininity at the same time. And my masculine and feminine urges are in complete agreement when they say to smash that box."

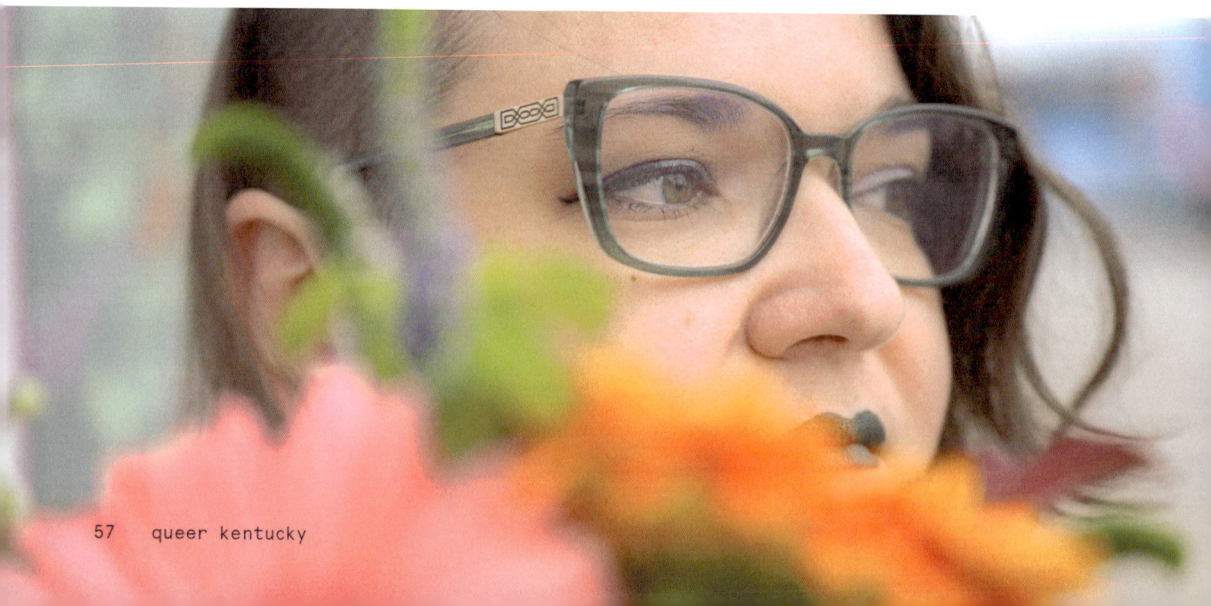

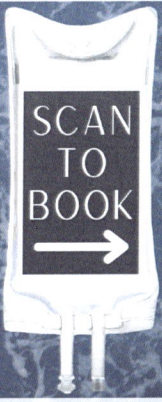

ETERNITY ⚭ WELLNESS

SCAN TO BOOK →

- IV HYDRATION TREATMENTS
- VITAMIN INJECTIONS
- INFRARED SAUNA
- BOTOX & FILLER
- HYDRAFACIAL & CRYOFACIAL
- WELLNESS MEMBERSHIPS
- SCAN FOR FULL MENU!

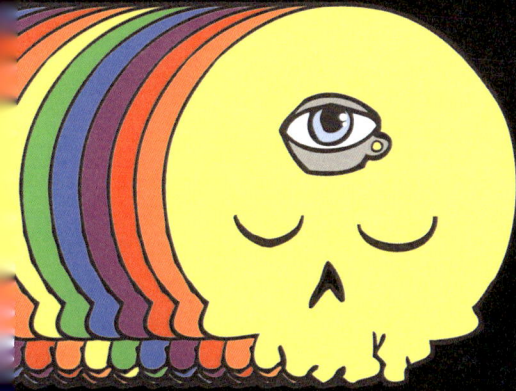

502.444.8100

LUSSI BROWN COFFEE BAR

EST. 2017

LUSSIBROWNCOFFEE.COM

Custom LogoWare

Certified LGBT

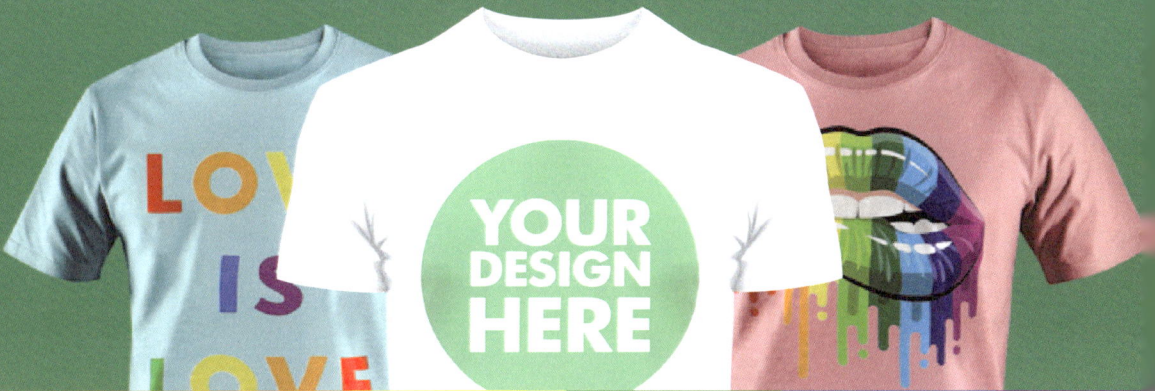

LOVE IS LOVE

YOUR DESIGN HERE

Custom Apparel & Branded Promotional Items

www.CustomLogoWa

Paper Cut Illustrations

Jack Manion *he/him* *@jackmanion*

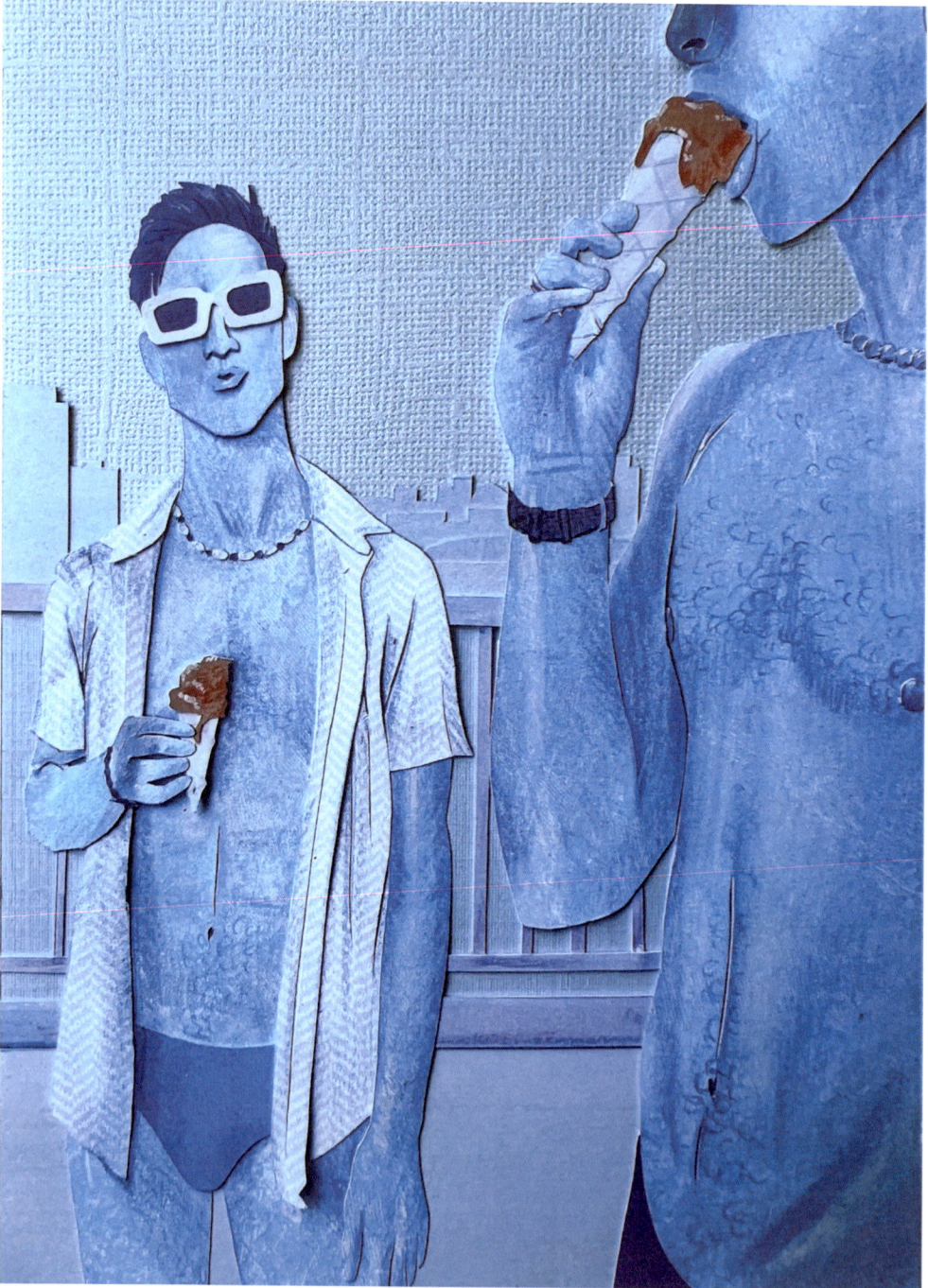

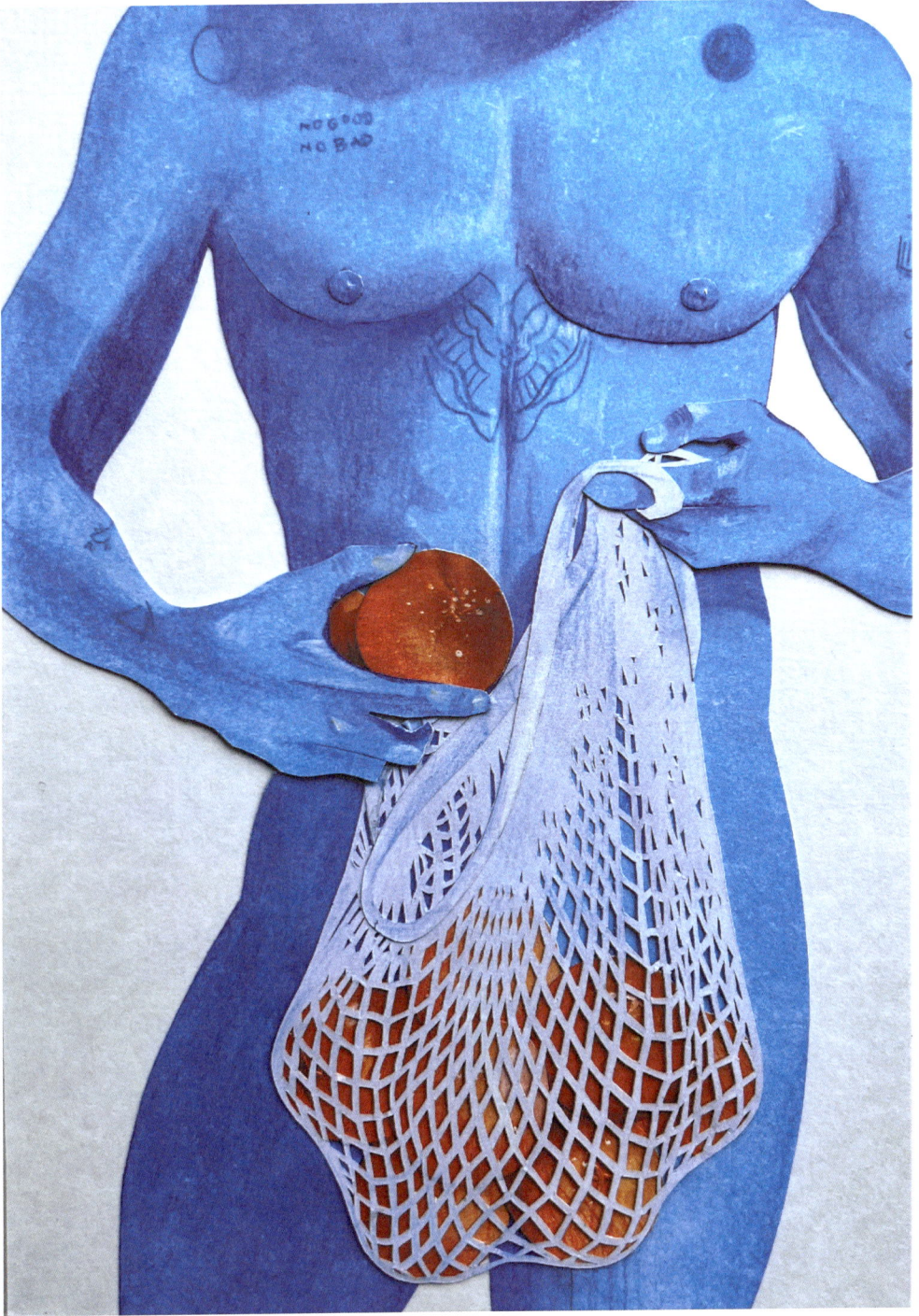

LOUISVILLE PRIDE FOUNDATION APPOINTS EXECUTIVE DIRECTOR

Tom Lally *he/him* *@tomlallyky*

The Louisville Pride Foundation hired an Executive Director who aims to make the Louisville Pride Center more accessible for the entire community, including people of all ages, folks in recovery, and people across the metro.

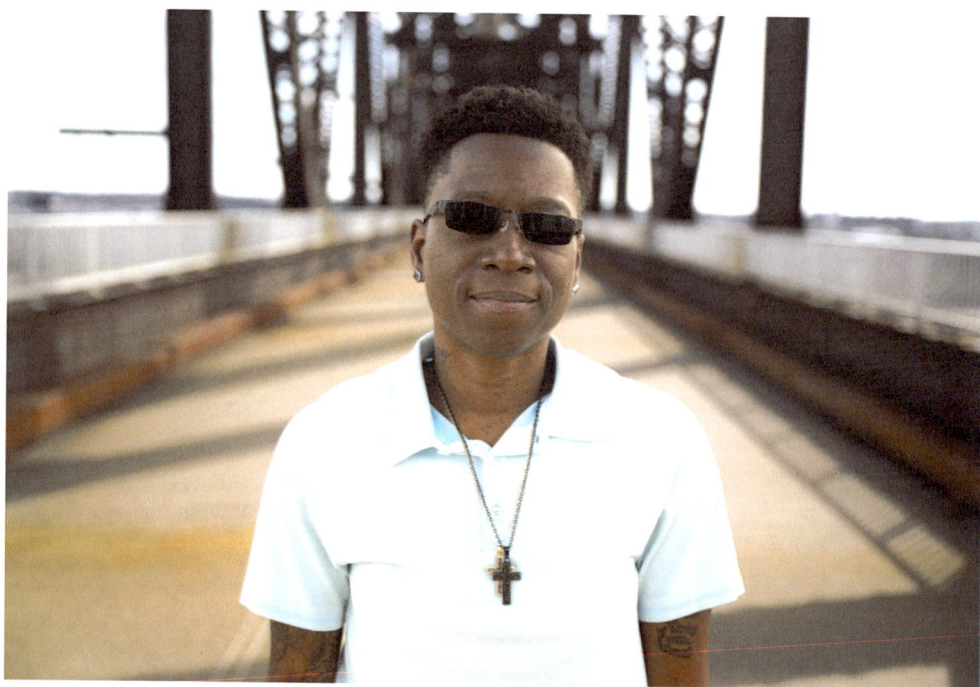

In December, the Louisville Pride Foundation's executive director, Mike Slaton, stepped down from his position to take a job with the Louisville Orchestra.

Ebony Cross, a Black and masculine-presenting woman, took on the new role of executive director entering 2024. Cross aims to prioritize representation through staff, events, and programing at the foundation and the Louisville Pride Center.

"Being a Black masculine or aggressive presenting woman in my new role is something I take great pride in and is an enormous opportunity. I don't take my role and responsibility lightly," Cross explained. In this new role, Cross is particularly interested in engaging queer people who live west of 9th Street, ensuring the pride center is a well-used resource for all neighbors in the Louisville metro.

That note strikes a chord with advocates across Louisville, including Chris Hartman. The Executive Director of the Fairness Campaign highlighted Louisville and Kentucky's lack of historical representation of Black and masculine-presenting women and the underlying positive impact her presence will have in this new role. "It's exciting to see where Ebony will take the important work of the Louisville Pride Foundation," Hartman said. "And it's incredibly important that other Black queer community members will see Ebony in this leadership role. Ebony will bring experiences and perspective that are historically underrepresented in our queer rights movement, and Louisville, our community, and the Pride Foundation will be better for it."

Originally from Akron Ohio, Ebony Cross followed love to Louisville more than a decade ago. Like most people in the 2010s, Cross was online dating and hoping to find someone special. It didn't take long; after back-and-forth messages, a first phone call and then a year of dating, Cross moved to Louisville's West End to live with their soon-to-be wife.

That love manifested and grew from one person to an entire community. Cross recalled a fascination with the people and places that make Louisville home, from Muhammad Ali to the Chickasaw Park, as well as its thriving queer community.

In September of 2022, Slaton successfully recruited Cross to join the Louisville Pride Foundation as an administrative coordinator. "What he did was absolutely wonderful, because none of this would have happened without him," Cross shared, reflecting on Slaton's initial and continued support. "He knew that leaving the foundation and the center in my hands - just in terms of growth and my vision and where I want to take it - he knew that was a great move."

The Louisville Pride Foundation also made history with its recent appointment of Victoria Syimone as Board Chair. A powerful performer and DJ, Syimone brings her experience as a Black trans woman born and raised in the River City to an increasingly representative organization for Louisville's LGBTQ+ community. Her team celebrates her confrontational spirit and commitment to educating and empowering our neighbors. In this new role, Cross is looking to change things.

Accessibility and representation are key themes in Cross's plan for the Louisville Pride

Foundation and Pride Center.

"Currently, we are open just two days out of the week... I would like to change that to be open to Monday through Friday," Cross shared. "So, we can kind of just keep that rotating foot traffic, you get the resources, you get the education, you can attend the events, you can book a space."

Cross also plans to build on existing programming, opening the door for youth and adults. The Foundation currently runs a harm reduction program to educate and empower members of the LGBTQ+ community on issues relating to drug use. Cross said they are also in the process of establishing new resources for community members who are food insecure, as well as an "immunity in the community" program promoting vaccination in urban and rural communities.

Cross takes on this new role at a difficult time for queer and trans people in the state of Kentucky. With new anti-trans laws banning gender-affirming care and a slew of newly introduced bills targeting diversity, equity and inclusion, the leader of a Pride Foundation in the Commonwealth's largest city bears the responsibility of not only supporting their immediate community, but also queer and trans people across the state.

"As long as we exist, and we are here, there's always going to be a message of hope," Cross promised.

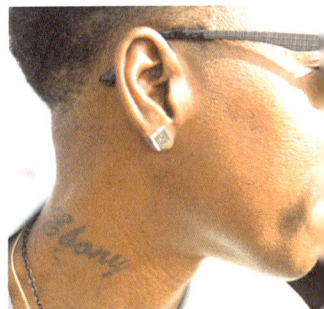

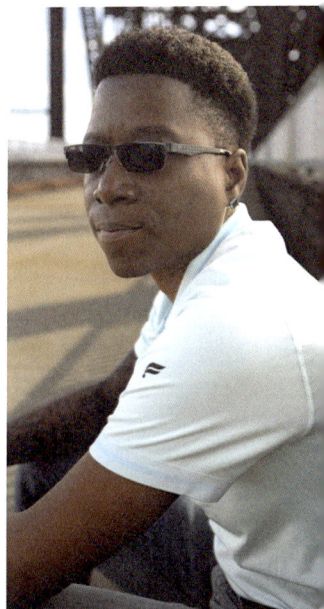

BRINGING UP BOYSLUT

DISCOVERING A SHAMELESS ROLE MODEL AS A BI BOI IN THE BLUEGRASS

BY SHEPHERD *he/they   @shepherdahlers*

I remember the first time I encountered Zachary Zane's bawdy reporting on the internet. I was searching for something that could help me make sense of my sexual identity.

His shameless approach to writing about sex horrified me at first. One such story graced my Instagram feed during a distracted moment at work. I felt my face flush red. This was decidedly the kind of material that launched NSFW as a daring acronym, and here I was, risking it all, to read descriptions of men gathering in a dark church for a ritual of giving and receiving anonymous bareback loads.

A sacrament like this was precisely the kind of blasphemous activity that would call down hellfire and condemnation from the pulpits of my past life. I recalled my own (tightly clenched) butthole alighting the pews of a different dark church for an endless string of Sundays, begging sky daddy to forgive me for thinking about such things, and liking it! Who exactly would Jesus do? I unfollowed.

Reading this aptly titled memoir, *Boyslut*, several years later, I realized I was too quick to shut down my curiosity. I recognize that my horror was precisely because I saw my own potential in Zane's ability to live shamelessly. My desire for my own sexual freedom lay smothered beneath a mask of inoffensive masculine acceptability that I adopted to keep me safe.

Zane describes the problem I was facing succinctly. Men, queer and straight alike, have been mostly left out of the sex positivity movement. The stakes were too high to not get this right, and we were suffering heartache, confusion, and disillusionment as a result.

He was on a parallel journey, writing about fucking in order to "unfuck" himself, in the best way possible.

Unlike me, and statistically a good many of you, Zane is keen to explain that he wasn't fucked up by religion. In fact his family was decidedly queer positive and affirming. And yet the messages of shame that were all too familiar to my experience, had marked his story from an early age. He puts it succinctly; "I can sum up my years of writing with one insight: I am not special."

It seems very few of us make it through childhood sufficiently unashamed of ourselves.

I was 14 when my father's interrogation of my most shameful secret (looking at porn on the family iMac) ended with his satisfaction that "at least I know you are not gay". What a relief that must have been for him. But I was brewing with a new set of fears – what if I was gay? Clearly to be gay was one of the worst things my father could imagine for his son.

Fear of coloring outside the wrong lines hid from me the romantic interest I had in male friends. I knew I was different. I didn't know

"IT'S A BOOK THAT READS AS A HOW-TO GUIDE, OR A DECENTLY AFFORDABLE STARTER PACK FOR BEING BISEXUAL IN THE WAY THAT SEEMS BEST TO YOU."

to know what kind of different I was. Looking back I recognize that I was awestruck by people who didn't meet gendered expectations. Even as a youngster I recall crushing on Bernard the elf from The Santa Clause. (This character still does it for me; he's forever the template.)

Much like Zachary, it took a lot of years of soul searching and misguided counsel before reaching a lightbulb moment. And just like him, my first exploration of my homoromantic side was an encounter with a serial manipulator. But despite added baggage, I learned something about myself definitively as a result. I liked being desired by a man, and I was into sucking cock–was it possible I wanted something more?

Unlike the stopover theory of bisexuality suggests, I didn't find this knowledge made me question my passion for the fairer sex (We can re-visit this phrase now that we have all seen Jacob Elordi wearing wings in Saltburn, right? Men can be downright angelic creatures!).

If I can truly fall in love with a person of any gender, how would I ever choose a "side" without feeling I was denying a significant part of myself, leaving it unexplored, or forever questioned?

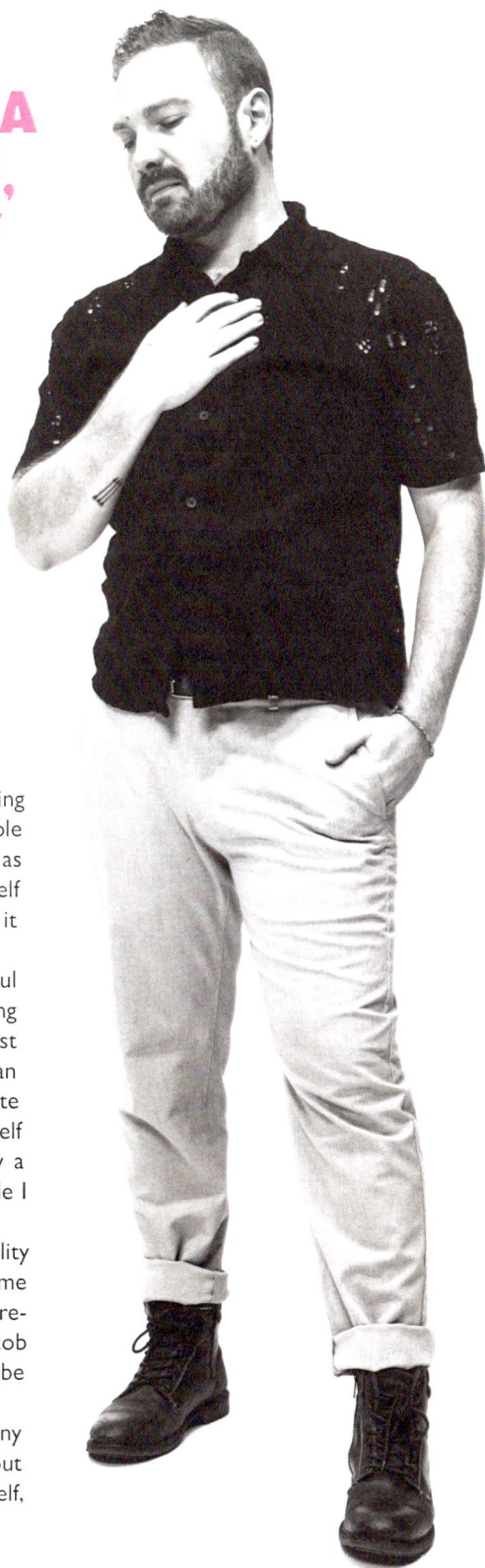

Zane argues that bisexual visibility is a misnomer. In untangling the messiness of the gay and straight cultural divide, he posits we adopt "bisexual audibility." Being vocal about our experiences allows others the opportunity to find a vocabulary for their own experiences too.

The stories he shares bring home the tenderness that surrounds what one might find a more "sordid" or "bohemian" lifestyle. Zane makes a great case that radical honesty and acceptance opens up possibilities for connection in far more satisfying ways than we might think. In choosing a polyamorous lifestyle, he was able to discover a world of dynamic and supportive relationships with men, women, and non-binary hotties, each with something unique and enticing to share. For Zane, it is a natural fit for a horny bisexual to want to have it all - and perhaps it is a bit greedy, but so what? It's not taken for granted here that this isn't everyone's desire, but this is *Boyslut* after all, and that means giving the best shot to having an open heart, as well as open holes.

This stuff is the author at his best. He has stories to share and a life well lived to pull from. The invitation and challenge is laid on the reader to push back against pervasive sex negativity with genuine joy and vulnerability.

The amount of second guessing, self doubt, and shame I have put myself through to date could easily fill out a memoir far less enlightening or entertaining as this book. The pages amount to a celebration of shameless, liberated, non-toxic masculinity. It's a book that reads as a how-to guide, or a decently affordable starter pack for being bisexual in the way that seems best to you.

AND IF ZACHARY ZANE IS BRAVE ENOUGH TO SPARK A BOYSLUT REVOLUTION WITH THE STROKES OF HIS PEN(IS), HE CAN AT THE VERY LEAST COUNT ME AMONG HIS FOLLOWING ONCE AGAIN.

Shepherd is a filmmaker in Louisville, KY.

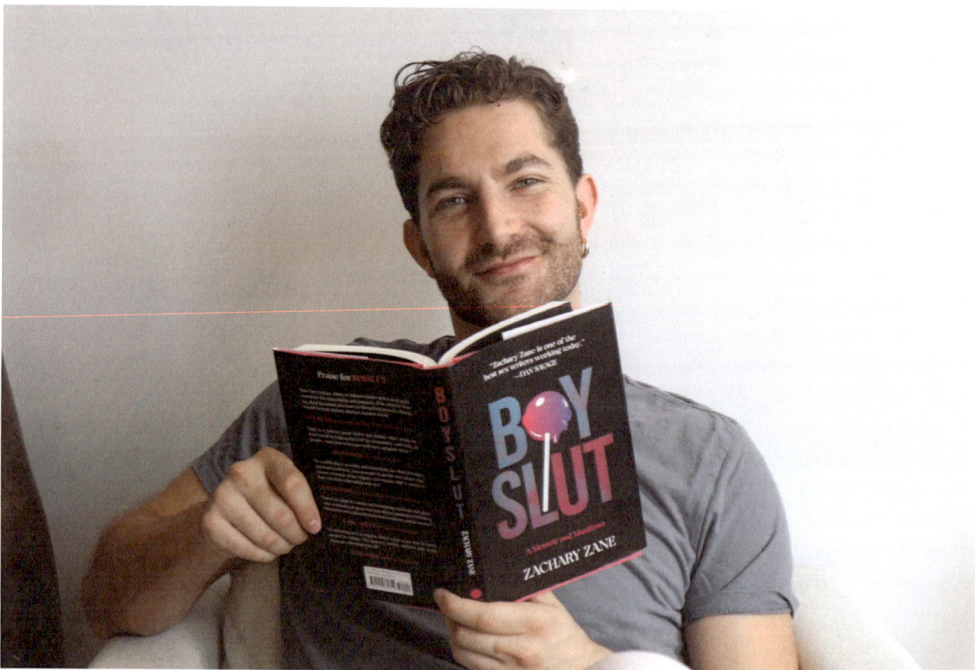

ZACHARY ZANE   *he/him*   *@zacharyzane_*

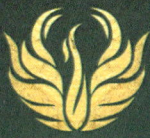

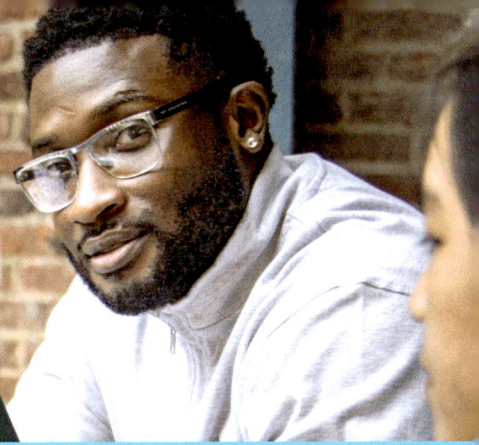

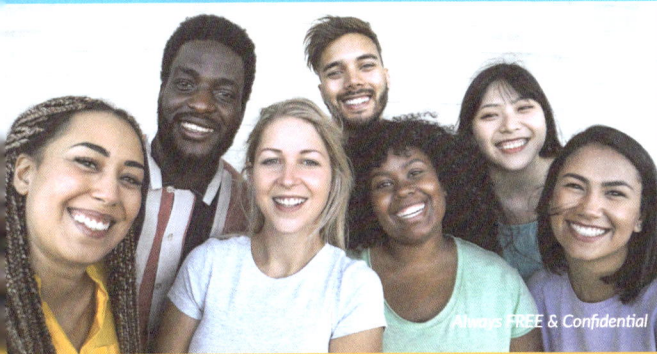

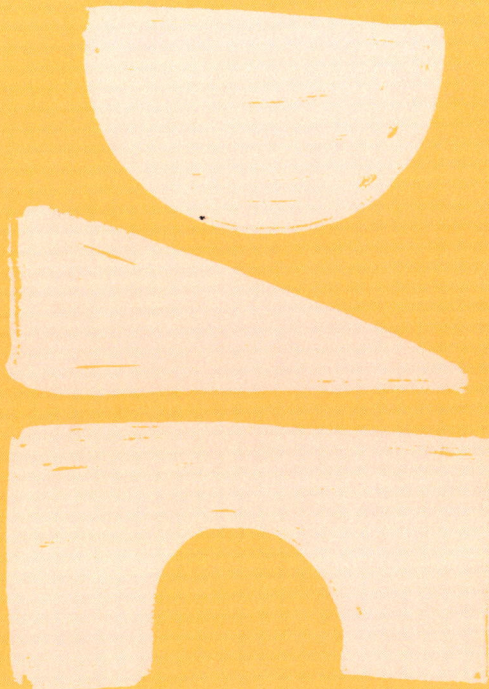

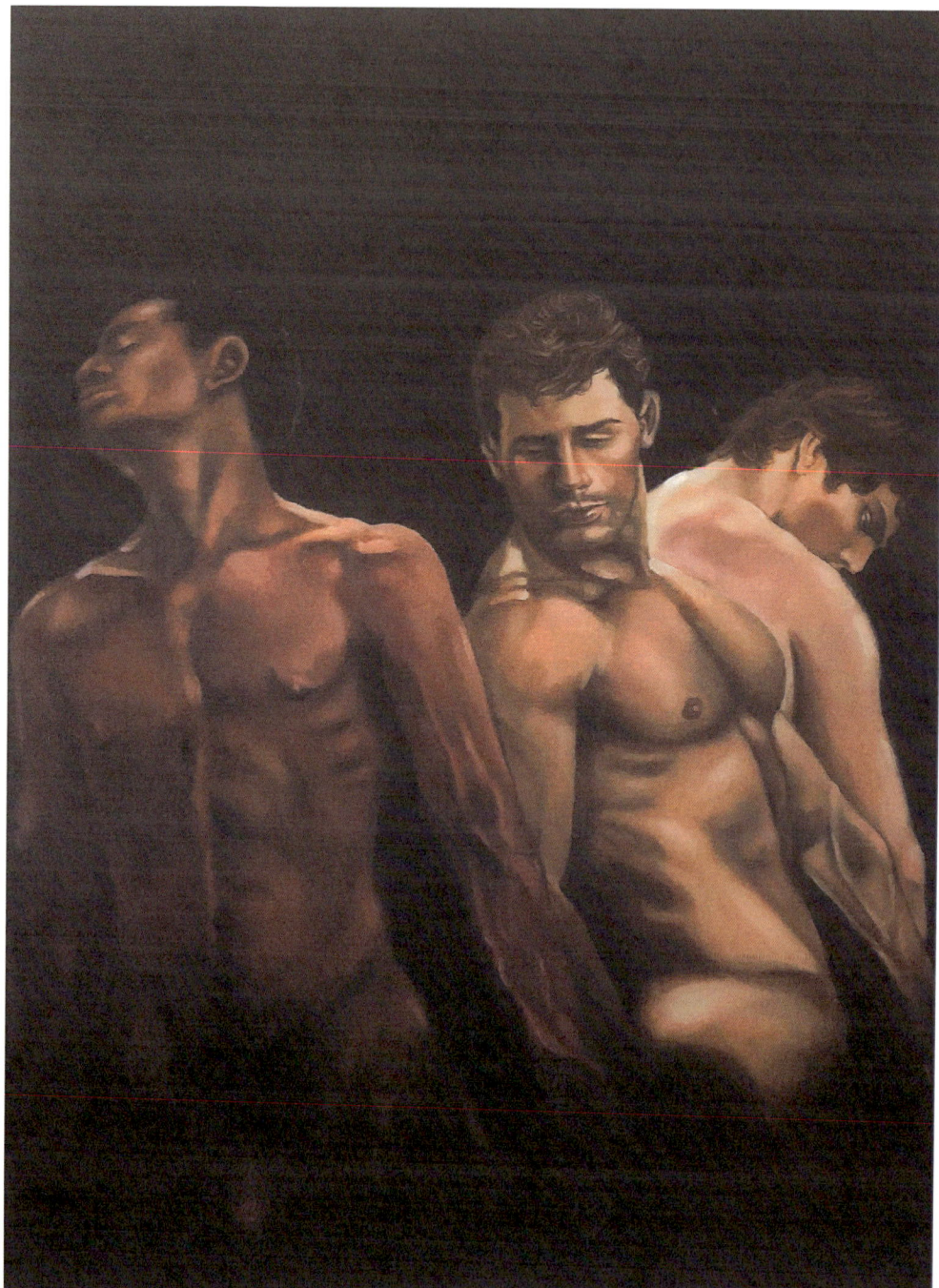

MASCULINITIES IN ART: CONSIDERING THE "OTHER"

Jacob Grant *he/him* *@jgartworks*

I struggle with understanding my own masculinity. Constantly, I am reminded in passing of my physical "unmanliness" whether it be in regards to my style of choice or how my attention to more feminine beauty regimens. I am not ashamed of these virtues; rather curious. As an openly gay artist, I look to investigate these relational qualities of the "to be or not to be" masculine, attempting to reexamine this concept through my own experiences as a cisgender male in heteronormative structures of society. Because I do not portray the typical physical attributes of a 'man'– tough, athletic, stoic– I am perceived as an "other." Albeit, such binaries ignore my traits of what I know establishes my maleness: adventure seeking, courage, gut feeling.

Recent artistic projects of mine probe this "other" maleness that is inappropriately represented within Kentuckian (albeit Western) Culture. To find success in such work, my most bold points are concealed within hidden symbolism and retrospect. In my work *Three Damn Figures*, 2023, the roles of these subjects retain ambivalent depictions of the masculine. The individuals are referenced from Gay Photographer David Vance's *Untitled (Three Men with Vines)*, c. 1990. A portion of his creative work involves the expression of gay desire and eroticism. Three Men with Vines depicts three figures who solemnly guard themselves behind a twisting vine that seems to pull a nature-esque background into fruition. Their gazes direct elsewhere from each other's own bodies, almost sensing a slight glance towards the other. In my piece, I use a thick, black oil paint base to create an abyss around these characters, spotlighting them as my target. While alienated, I avert fragments of their bodies, allowing the spotlight to linger. When considering what masculinity is, there is little aesthetic responsibility when depicting the male simulacrum. Likewise, my piece does not offer that narrative, settling for a flux between physical perception and self actualization.

As I continue painting and dissecting these concepts I realize the "other" is still being legitimized. However, the masculine is a basic, performative idea of what engenders these characteristics. I've naively correlated the "other" to a concept of Hybrid Masculinity (a term expounding R.W. Connell's critical role theory of hegemonic and subordinate masculinities). This theory was criticized by the theoretician Demetrakis Z. Demetriou (2001) for its rigidity. He posits that hybrid masculinities demystify contemporary inequalities present between genders and race; they are not categorized. Demetriou's most notable critique is that it resolves to agency, ill grasping of the culturally masculine ideal. In whitewashed gay communities, the standard hegemonic masculine type is repurposed as the ideal, whereas the other groups suffer from ostracization: Am I too feminine? Am I too skinny or too fat for my body to be desired? Could wealth indicate I have triumphed against a Queer-Exclusionist society? Does inherent masculinity exclude individuals of other gender identities?

These theories are the basic frameworks for understanding masculinity, though I suggest re-examining these dialogues to be substantial. There remains in that emerging dialogue a radical queer potential to realize. Considering Queer Futurity, José Esteban Muñoz recalls a then and there perspective to imagine the untouchable, perfect existence of queerness. The "to be or not to be" masculine does not exist-unless is truly performative. However, the "other" will persist, especially if society chooses to absolve itself of holding masculinity to a binary. As a fragment of my work, *Three Damn Figures* is my method of traversing along the "could be(s)" of queer embodiment. I do believe hybrid masculinity does not encourage conversations of this "other." I wish to dissolve the meaning of the body and examine the fundamentals of how maleness is conceived as masculine. Admittedly, masculinity is an engendered characteristic that might not need to be reimagined. Rather, it should be realized as it belongs to various types of people who identify with the term. Isn't that what queerness begs us to think forward to? I realize as I continuously try to poke and pry at this idea through my work, I am dissolving what I have thought masculinity means in our culture. This "other" masculine may be a curtain pulled down to glimpse towards a direction of ungendered experience and identity. And still, I am other.

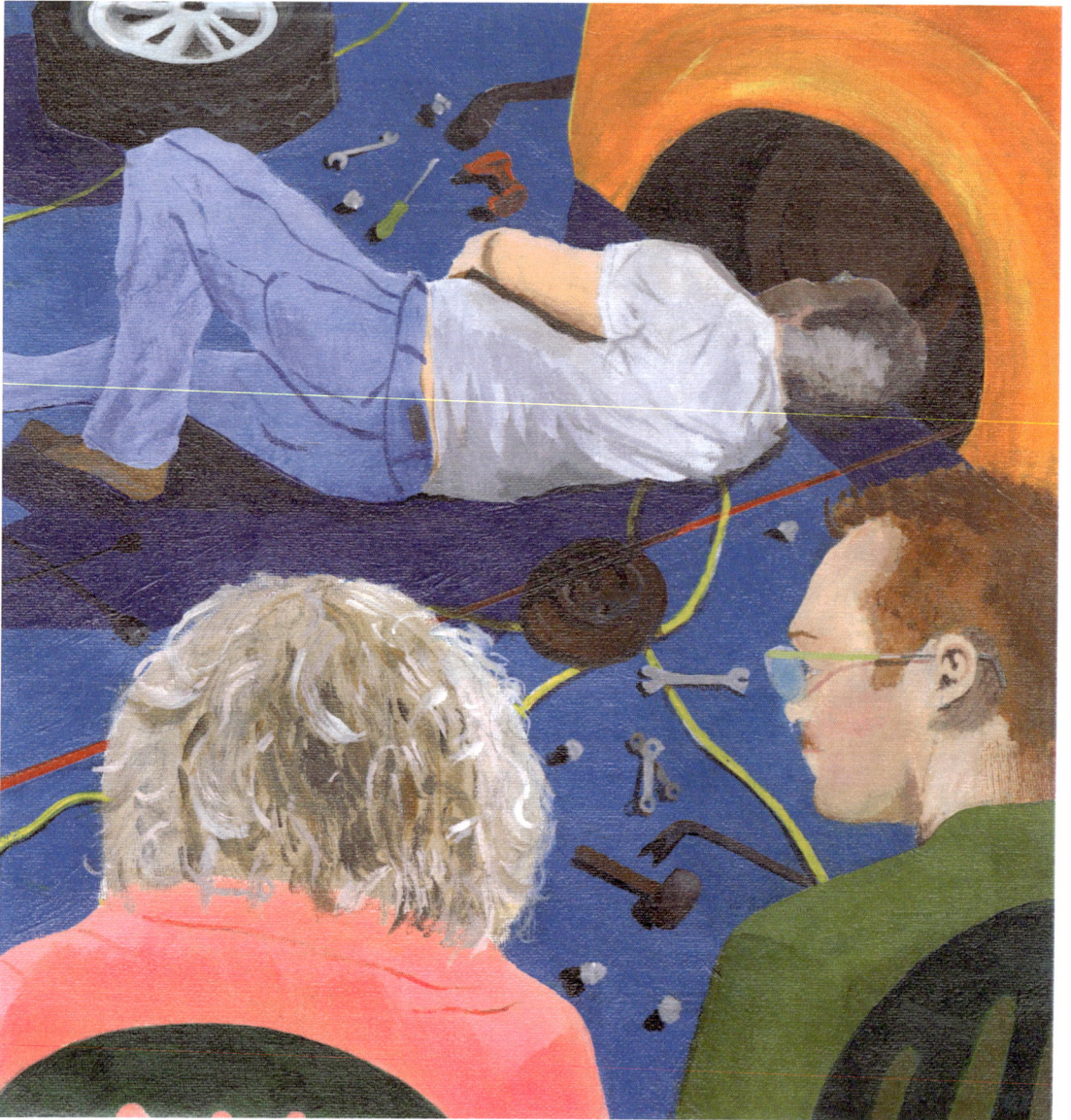

TRANSMISSION

Levi House   *he/him*   *@arthous3*

As a trans man, I've been asking myself for years what it means to be a man and to be masculine. This is one of the things that led me to creating this piece, which originated from the time my car broke down and my grandfather became determined to fix it.

Upon his declaration to get to work, I offered my assistance, but my grandparents had other plans in mind: my papaw, in his stubborn old country man way, had resolved to make the complicated repair totally on his own. My mamaw decided she and I were going to help in a way I didn't expect.

We pulled up two green plastic lawn chairs a ways away from my grandfather, close enough to hear the frustrations under his breath, clicking of his teeth as he discarded tool after tool, but far enough away to make him feel like he had plenty of space. This left room for us to have our own private conversation.

We sat, observing quietly, then started gabbing. It felt at first like we were all just there with each other, but as I continued to periodically assert my availability to help Papaw between conversations with Mamaw, I realized there was a divide. There was him: the fixer, the holder of things, the determiner of tools, the carrier of the burden and reward of repair. Then, there was us: the girlies, gossiping, waiting for the big guns to finish the job, sent to the sidelines by the VIP.

That's how it seemed, until mid-gab, when Papaw almost dropped the car jack on himself and before anyone could realize the danger, Mamaw swooped in to save him from the threat.

She made her move, to the annoyance and resistance of my tired and irritable grandpa, and gracefully returned to her stoop alongside me in the girlies' green lawn chairs.

It became clear to me after that—she understood.

She understood that my grandfather would reject any help offered, but that he would need it and when he did, she would see it. She would be there, ready to take action, without even a moment's notice.

This is what masculinity feels like to me. It feels like looking at the options and tools available, hoping one will fit, learning what works, discarding what doesn't. Sometimes it's using the available tools to make more tools, more options, and hoping that what you build is useful to and works for the rest of the world.

This scene and masculinity both make me think about the divides that exist between masculine and feminine people; the spaces that masculine people are given that often overextend themselves into or overshadow spaces that feminine people are in, and can determine how much space feminine people are even allowed to take up. I think about how masculine people are so often highlighted in the foreground, but how even if we aren't allowed to see it, there are always feminine people that are doing the work: the essential work, the skilled but unappreciated labor.

I think about how often masculinity comes out of a sort of "knowing" – how when two men are moving a hefty, awkward sofa, there is an unspoken rule where they should just "know" where to go, anticipate where the other person is going, and move gracefully with the other to accomplish the goal in this totally silent, but still somehow communicated way.

I think about how my grandma knew that any outside help – especially from a woman or a young trans man who knows next to nothing about cars – would not be accepted, but was certain that at some point assistance would be imperative. Because she knew this, she made her silent plan to work in the way she knew it needed to.

I have been on T for six years now, which has made me super cis-passing. As my transition has progressed, the way I've been treated by both men and women has exponentially changed. When I greet men like I would anyone else, with a smile and a quick "howdy," sometimes it comes out a little too jolly or rushed and I can instantly see a look of assessment. It is such a fragile thing. Even one small inflection can be passed over as a judgment of "too feminine," or "weird," or "not man enough."

Recently, my downstairs neighbors found out I'm queer. The two housemates were always polite and minded their business aside from a courteous "hey man" in passing. Once, after I walked a date out the door, kissed him, and came back inside, I caught them looking out the window underneath the curtain at me, which they had never done before. After that, neither of them ever said hello to me again.

This is clearly a case of homophobia, but isn't homophobia rooted in toxic masculinity, too? The boys look at me different because I'm gay, but also because with that notion, they see less than. They see not man enough, fairy, faggot.

I have spent years trying to assess my own relationship to masculinity as a trans man with most of my life lived as a woman. I have learned that I think it's all kind of bullshit, but it's also kind of beautiful— the times when you do greet another man with a polite "howdy" that maybe comes out "too sweet" and it's received with a welcoming smile and a "howdy" back. The times that I've been smoking a cigarette at a coffee shop, looking feminine as hell, nails painted dark green, earrings in, all pink fit, legs crossed, and still another boy, a stranger, approaches me and asks if he can join me smoking my cigarette, and nothing we talk about is related to who we are or how we show up in the world, and then, a bond forms because we are both boys. The times that I hang out with my trans masc friend, the first trans boy I ever met who was my age, and we talk about the different parts of being a trans masc person, how to stick to our values and stick up for ourselves and other people in a world that makes it really scary to do so, bond-

I think: maybe masculinity is not just a look; it's a way of being, of feeling, of living.

ing over the shared horrors of men's restrooms, the dreams of an all-trans-led auto shop called "Transmission," and dreams of a world where trans people are part of the norm and you don't have to be passing to be seen as who you are.

I've spent all this time asking myself, "what is masculinity? What does it mean to be masculine?" and there are so many parts that feel so good and so right, but there are just as many parts that feel so foreign and wrong. I still can't totally put my finger on all the different moving parts, but I know that masculine is something I am. It's something that feels flexible to me, malleable and living, and it's also unique to every person – even if it might not seem like that on the surface.

When I am in spaces where I'm super aware I'm a masculine person where I can sometimes feel like I'm perceived as a threat, or I'm in spaces with a lot of other masculine people where I sometimes feel challenged because of my own toxic masculinity and wanting to prove myself as "man enough," I think of situations like this with my grandparents where there is a lot to take in, unpack, and learn from.

I think: maybe masculinity is not just a look; it's a way of being, of feeling, of living.

It's my papaw making it his priority to take care of me, maybe in a way that showcases his masculinity, but not just because he wants to show off, because he wants it done right, because he has the experience to make him confident that he can do so, because he believes the least he can do is try to be there. It's my mamaw having seen the situation enough times to know she'll have to be strategic and stay on the sidelines until the time to interject that she knows will come. It's me watching it all, assessing and learning, inventorying for my next session of wondering and trying hard to keep all of the discoveries and notes with me the next time I act.

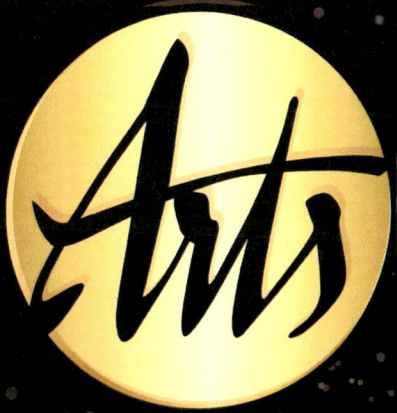

75 YEARS

IN THE

CITY OF

ARTISTS

CELEBRATE WITH US AT
FUNDFORTHEARTS.ORG

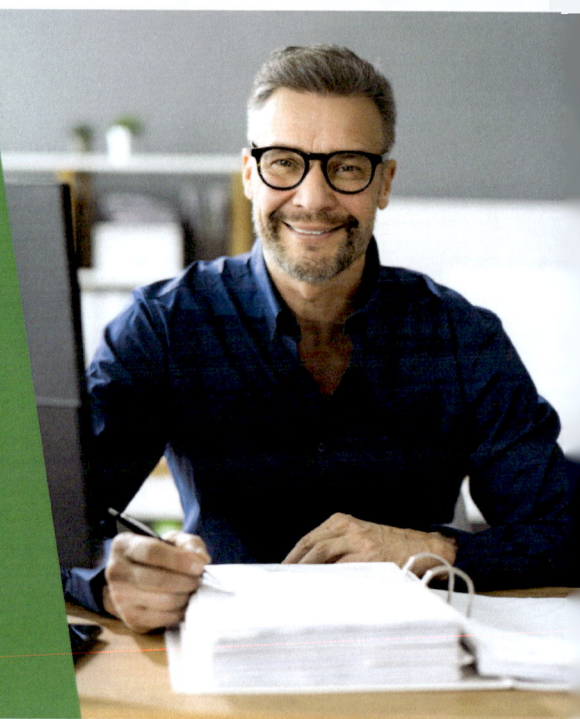

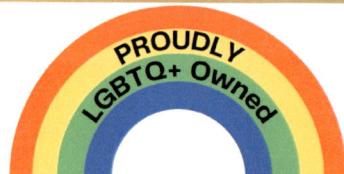

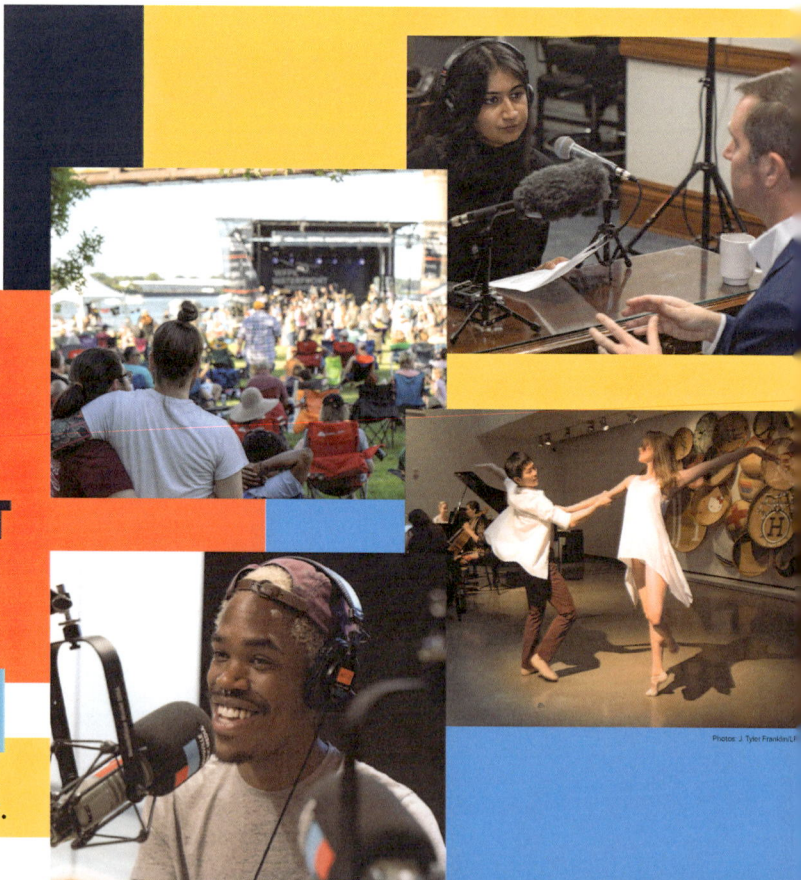

www.ingramcontent.com/pod-product-compliance
Lightning Source LLC
Chambersburg PA
CBRC101145030426
42337CB00009B/74